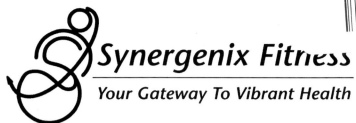

Synergenix Fitness
Your Gateway To Vibrant Health

Presents the

Healthy Habit Former

A 90-day Self-directed Action Plan
for those who want a
Calm Mind & Vibrant Body

A gift for

_____

You are receiving this program because
I care about your health and wellbeing.

Signed _____

Special Thanks

I would like to thank the following colleagues and friends
who have contributed to the success of this project:
Bill Bartmann, Dr. Michael Jones, Dan Barton, Michael Losier,
T. Harv Eker, Ted Roberts, Dr. Brian Walsh, Dr. Brian Pound.

Disclaimer

**Synergenix Fitness recommends that you obtain your doctor's
approval before beginning this program.** Your doctor may have
specific recommendations for you to follow regarding various aspects
of the program.

Each person is unique. Throughout this program, it is important that
you participate only in the activities that you feel are right for you.
The author believes that the information presented in this program is
sound; however, *Synergenix Fitness* and the author cannot be held
responsible for either the actions participants take or the result of
their actions. Each person is responsible for any and all actions in
which they engage.

If you feel unsure about anything, it is your responsibility to seek
professional advice/help before proceeding.

By beginning the **Healthy Habit Former** *program*, you agree to the
conditions outlined above.

Contact us

Astrid Whiting,
www.SynergenixFitness.com
Astrid@SynergenixFitness.com
Victoria, BC, Canada

To place an order for bulk copies of the **Healthy Habit Former**,
or to enquire about speaking engagements please contact
Synergenix Fitness at 250-888-4099.

Contents

What others are saying

At every turn, Astrid incorporates the Law of Attraction in her *Healthy Habit Former* program. Each activity in the book is designed to have you put "energy, attention, and focus" on creating healthy habits. Her daily activities get you to focus on "what you do want". For creating a healthy active lifestyle, her program is the Law of Attraction in action.

Michael Losier, bestselling author of *Law of Attraction*

I must say......FANTASTIC!!! The development of the fitness habit is so vitally important. The *Healthy Habit Former* is exactly the right tool for anyone wanting to embark on a fitness/health program that will really work! This program is safe, simple and incorporates highly effective coaching techniques. By following this program to the letter the only possible outcome is a healthy, active lifestyle! Astrid has created a tool that has long been needed in the fitness industry and I highly recommend her Workbook.

Michael K. Jones PhD, President,
American Academy of Health, Fitness, and Rehabilitation Professionals

Astrid's approach to personal training is an asset to the industry and a breath of fresh air. She has created an easy to follow program that could service the immediate needs of individuals challenged with integrating daily exercise into their schedules.

Kathi Cameron, Kinesiologist, School of Physical Education,
University of Victoria

Thank you so much for the *Healthy Habit Former* Workbook. I am so energized and excited...what the workbook does, using clear writing, simple advice, and a holistic approach, is give me a day-to-day, step-by-step process to get fit, and stay that way. I love that you have positive self-image built into the program. I have been reading the book to my kids at the breakfast table, and already they are living by the chant "raw, raw, raw!". I am thrilled about this, because if the workbook can instill healthy habits in myself, AND also in my kids, then wow, what incredible value. Thank you, again.

Gerry Brimacombe, President, Sector Learning, Victoria BC

I just received my Workbook... It seems simple enough and significant in how it affects the most critical areas of our lives - thank you for your work!

Sandi Borgmeyer, Mary Kay Cosmetics, Menomonie, WI

I am a man who knows something about success, and failure. I have gone through many ups and downs on my way to becoming a billionaire, and one thing I have learned is there is no substitute for a proven system. Effort without knowledge of how something works and/or a concrete plan to accomplish it is a waste of energy.

This is true in business and it's true for your health. When you have a proven system, stick with it and you will reach all of your goals. Out of knowledge and experience Astrid has put together a concrete system, that when followed, will lead to certain success in creating a healthy, active life-style. The *Healthy Habit Former* hands to you on a platter a plan that works. Use it, and be successful!

Bill Bartmann, author of *Billionaire Secrets To Success*

Proper nutrition is vital to good health. In her book the *Healthy Habit Former* Astrid provides users an easy to follow template that will create very nourishing, and healthy eating habits. Combined with the other components in her program, this action plan provides the user a solid foundation of overall health, and wellness.

Adam Hart, Whole Foods Personal Trainer,
Director and Founder of Clear Impact Consulting Inc.

In her *Healthy Habit Former* program, Astrid masterfully incorporates accelerated teaching techniques with simple, easy-to-do daily activities. These elements create an amazing synergy that will accelerate your results. What a concept. There is no other program that contains such a powerful combination.

Brian E Walsh PhD, bestselling author of *Unleashing Your Brilliance*

Astrid has put together a program that everyone can benefit from. There is something here that can fit into everyone's lifestyle, in a comfortable, effective, and ease of use manner. We are all fortunate to have some of her expertise shared and available.

Gregg Turner BA CHT CNLT CTT, International Wellness Consultant,
Public Appointee to the College of Naturopathic Physicians of BC

Wow, Astrid! I believe this is a first of its kind. What you have succeeded in doing here is to provide a very balanced program, that is easy to follow, based on very reliable theory. You have provided a workbook that will fit everyone's time schedule and make it easy to complete. The idea of creating new habits provides benefits that will last a life time.

Dr. Brian Pound MB BS LRCP MRCS LMCC   1.05

A Welcome Message from Astrid

Welcome, and congratulations on your decision to create healthy, active habits. A lot of people *talk* about creating a healthier lifestyle, but few actually do anything about it. You, on the other hand, are different. By obtaining, the **Healthy Habit Former** 90-day self-directed action plan, you have separated yourself from the "all talk/ no action" crowd. You have taken that important first step towards creating a healthier, active lifestyle. Well done!

The purpose of this program is to assist you to reprogram yourself so that healthy, active lifestyle choices become habitual. Creating new habits is a process, but I guarantee that if you follow this program, day-by-day, step-by-step, you will absolutely create healthy, active lifestyle habits.

> *Ninety-five percent of your behavior is a result of patterns and habits.*
>
> *The more a person performs any new skill, the stronger the habit becomes.*
>
> Dr. Brian Walsh

We are creatures of habit. Some habits serve us, others don't.

Most people believe that it takes 21 to 30 days to establish a new pattern or habit. Actually, recent research tells us that you can establish a new habit in as little as 5 days. Now, here's the catch – the old habit is still there; desperately holding on to its turf. Every time you practice the new habit, it gets stronger, and the old habit begins to weaken. Of course the opposite is true - every time you revert to the old habit, it gains profile and strength, and the new habit begins to fade.

Your choice is simple. Since you want to establish new healthy habits, you must rehearse the new patterns as often as you can. How long will this take? Well, although simple patterns can be replaced in as little as 30 days, more complicated ones will require a longer period. Hypnotherapist Dr. Brian Walsh says, "Well-entrenched patterns, which have been built up over years, will most likely need three months to replace thoroughly."

The **Healthy Habit Former** program is specifically designed to release unproductive patterns, while solidly entrenching healthy, active lifestyle habits. This is why your action plan encourages you to engage in five meaningful activities everyday, for 90 days.

1.06

The daily actions in this program may seem simplistic, perhaps a little unusual, and some of the concepts may even be completely new to you. That's okay. This program utilizes powerful training principles and processes designed to accelerate your results. I'm going to ask you to trust the process, and follow the action plan to the letter, even if something feels a little new to you.

> **We are what we repeatedly do.**
>
> **Excellence then is not an act, but a habit.**
>
> Aristotle

As you progress through the program, I want you to go easy on yourself. The mind doesn't like change, even good change. Your mind may attempt to sabotage your efforts by telling you that the program isn't working, or that there isn't time each day to do the activities. It may tell you that some of the activities are silly or a waste of time. This is a common experience. It's just your mind being lazy, and not wanting to change it's programming to a new way of being, even if it is healthier! So if you notice your mind attempting to sabotage you, simply say out loud "Thanks for that, I'm doing this anyway" - and do an activity from your action plan immediately.

Consistency and regularity are important to your success in the program. I know you will do your best to stay committed to completing your activities each day.

Now, you and I both know that life happens, and sometimes unexpected events occur. If something throws you off, and you happen to get off track for a bit — *relax*. Just pick up where you left off the next day. It's okay, just keep going. I know you can do it.

About Synergenix Fitness

At *Synergenix Fitness*, we help people improve their physical and mental health. Using fitness as a doorway, we guide you to your inner strengths and unlimited potential. You are a magnificent being capable of so much more than you may currently believe. Our aim is to help you rediscover your inner greatness.

> **The size of your success**
> **is determined by the size of your beliefs.**
>
> David Schwartz

Meet Astrid

Astrid Whiting brings twenty-five years of competitive sports experience to her role as a fitness professional. She is a Certified Medical Exercise Specialist, a Certified Personal Trainer, and the owner of Synergenix Fitness.

She helps people reach their fitness goals through her popular audio program, *Achieve Your Vibrant Healthy Body*, her presentations, teleclasses, one-on-one coaching, and magazine columns.

As a professional trainer, Astrid has experience working with people from a variety of ages, backgrounds and abilities. She combines her sports experience, knowledge of the body, and use of accelerated coaching techniques to create a potent synergy that allows her to guarantee results with her clients.

She has helped her clients:
- *achieve their optimal body shape*
- *eliminate high blood pressure medications*
- *feel fitter and stronger than they ever have*
- *reach personal bests in their sports*
- *regain total pain-free function in joints after surgery*
- *perform physical feats they never though possible*
- *regain their self-confidence and self-assuredness*
- *reverse Type 2 Diabetes*

1.08

Benchmark

Before we begin the program, let's take a quick assessment of your current lifestyle and attitudes. Please indicate the choice that best describes your current situation.

I currently exercise:

never   occasionally   In a week: 1 x   2 x   3 x   MORE

What role does exercise have in determining how you feel overall?

Not important   somewhat important   very important   essential

What is your current attitude towards exercise?

hate it   it's okay   enjoy it   love it

I eat raw fruits and vegetables:

never   occasionally   In a day: 1 x   2 x   3 x   MORE

I think raw fruits taste:

disgusting   okay   good   delicious

I think raw vegetables taste:

disgusting   okay   good   delicious

How would you describe your ability to calm and relax yourself?

very difficult   I can sometimes   I can most times   I can anytime

How do you feel about yourself and your current lifestyle?

not happy   somewhat happy   pretty happy   fantastic

You will be referring back to this page at the end of your program.   1.09

Notes

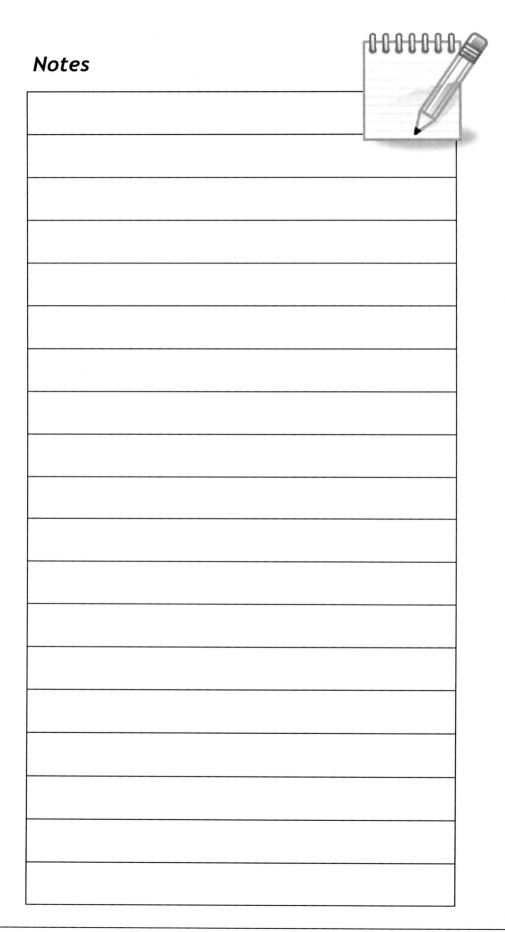

Workbook Instructions

In his book "*The Law of Attraction*", Michael Losier says, "We attract to our lives whatever we give our energy, attention or focus to." In other words, anytime we give attention to something, even just for a few minutes, the 'Law of Attraction' will automatically bring more of that into our lives.

I told you earlier that the **Healthy Habit Former** program uses many advanced training methodologies designed to accelerate your results. One of these techniques is to harness the powerful effects of the 'Law of Attraction'.

Each day you will be asked to perform five healthy activities. Some of these will be done each day, some once per week, and some done three times per week. Each time you spend a few minutes focusing on any activity in your action plan you will automatically be enlisting the 'Law of Attraction' which will obediently begin to compound what you are focusing on, thereby accelerating your results.

> *The groundwork of all happiness is health.*
>
> Leigh Hunt

An explanation of how and why to do each activity is outlined below.

Begin each day by opening up your Workbook, filling in the date, and completing the first activity. Then, simply read the remaining activities, incorporate them into your day, and log what you've done on your daily sheet.

Daily Activities:

Do these four activities everyday.
1. *Take five revitalizing breaths*
2. *Be active*
3. *Eat raw fruits and vegetables with every meal*
4. *Acknowledge yourself*

The fifth activity will be one of:
- *Three exercise sessions*
- *Four weekly acceleration tools*

Healthy Habit Former

1. Take 5 Revitalizing Breathes

We are all busy people. We fill our days with tasks, and stimulation from the moment we get up to the moment our head finally hits the pillow at night. Although this is becoming the expected societal norm, it is a dangerous practice, as we perpetually begin to live in a cycle of constant sensory input, and activity. This hurried, and stimulant-full lifestyle choice often leads to increased stress, inability to focus, short attention spans, emotional imbalance, high blood pressure, fear, poor eating and sleeping patterns, and strained relationships.

We require daily personal quiet time in order to feel calm and peaceful. A lot of people tell me they simply can't fit quiet time in for themselves. After all, they have to make meals, go to work or school, look after others, run errands, do chores, watch TV, and work on the computer. If they want to address the needs of their family, and work, there simply isn't time for self care. Well guess what? I'm here to tell you there is, and it is **vital**.

Would you do a better job at school or work when you are stressed and hurried, or when you are calm and at ease? Would you interact better with people you love when you are calm, or when you are racing to get a million things done? You know the answer as well as I do. So, the question is... *What are you going to do about it?*

> ### *Breathe... just breathe.*
> Lyrics from Anna Nalick

One solution is to begin habitually taking time to simply breathe. Rarely in our fast-paced world do we take the time to take in a long, deep breath. You know, one that really pushes out our tummy!

Deep breathing has been used for centuries to calm the body, quiet and sharpen the mind, accelerate healing, slow aging, and circulate oxygen-rich blood throughout the body to revitalize cells, and provide steady energy.

2.01

There are many different breathing patterns, and techniques. The technique you are going to use is called *square breathing*. Square breathing is excellent as it is particularly easy to learn, doesn't take much time, can be done anywhere, and is extremely effective. You'll be amazed how calm, and renewed this will make you feel.

To begin entrenching a habit of quiet time, each morning, I want you to do 5 revitalizing breath cycles. This will help you to start your day on a calm, clear note.

Each breath cycle will take 16 seconds.
- *Breathe in through your nose deeply for 4 seconds*
- *Hold that breath for 4 seconds*
- *Breathe out through your mouth for 4 seconds*
- *Hold for 4 seconds*
- *Repeat the cycle*

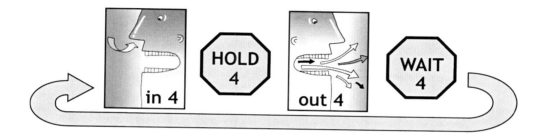

As you become more proficient at this technique, you may begin increasing the length of each breath cycle. Feel free to do more square breathing anytime during the day. Particularly if you feel tired, stressed, frazzled or rushed.

Healthy Habit Former

2. Be Active

Although we choose to be busier and busier, we are becoming more and more sedentary. We spend hours a day sitting in front of a computer, we use remotes instead of getting up to change the channel, we watch countless hours of TV. In the name of convenience, and saving time we order products online, have someone else make our coffee, take the elevator instead of the stairs, drive instead of walk, and we even have food delivered to our door. When was the last time you came home from work or school, got changed, and went outside for a while?

> *I still get wildly enthusiastic about little things...*
> *I play with leaves,*
> *I skip down the street, and run against the wind.*
>
> Leo Buscaglia

A sedentary lifestyle can creep up on you without you really realizing it. A sedentary lifestyle weakens your muscles, increases your weight, decreases circulation, taxes your heart, reduces energy, enables disease, and means more trips to health care professionals. The number of people with Type 2 Diabetes (*the totally preventable and reversible kind*) is the highest it's ever been in history! A sedentary lifestyle makes for a shorter, and poorer quality of life, period.

If you want to enjoy a vibrant quality of life, and be active and healthy well into your later years, you must to get back into a pattern of staying active *now*. Fortunately, this is very easy to do. It's all about your daily *choices*; something over which *you* have complete control.

> *A body at rest tends to stay at rest,*
> *and a body in motion tends to stay in motion.*
>
> Newton's law

To get back into a habitual cycle of active living, do at least one physical activity per day that you wouldn't normally do. For instance:

- *Dance around the house*
- *Go for a walk during your coffee or lunch break*
- *Learn to juggle*
- *Walk up the stairs rather then using the elevator*
- *Play Frisbee or lawn darts with a friend*
- *Walk to the store*
- *Go bowling or play pool*
- *Use an exercise ball as your desk chair*

Have fun with this. Be creative, and encourage others to do the same.

2.03

3. Raw, Raw, Raw
Eat Raw Fruits and Vegetables with Every Meal

Healthy living requires healthy foods. Food is the fuel your body uses for everything it does, such as brain functioning, healing, metabolizing, creating hormones, building bones, digesting, creating and maintaining muscle, ensuring chemical balance, and providing energy.

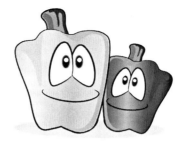

Unfortunately, as a society we are eating more and more processed foods. Have you looked around your grocery store lately? What percentage of the store is devoted to packaged food, compared to fresh, raw foods? Now, what about *your kitchen*?

The more we process (package) and cook food, the less value it has for our bodies. When we heat food we begin to destroy it's living enzymes. Processed food is routinely stripped of its naturally-occurring nutrients, and then impregnated with chemical ones. It's loaded with sugar, salt, artificial ingredients, and color. When we feed our body dead, unnatural, processed material, how can we possibly expect optimal performance?

Raw food is full of Mother Nature's finest ingredients. It contains living enzymes, natural vitamins, minerals, fiber, water, carbohydrates, and proteins, all designed to be easily and readily accepted by your body. If you want optimal health, and performance, give your body high-grade fuel. Give it "raw energy."

> *Never eat more than you can lift.*
>
> Miss Piggy

To get back into the habit of healthy eating, commit to eating raw fruits and/or vegetables with each meal. Do your best to <u>cover at least half of your plate </u>with fruits and/or vegetables, that are uncooked or un-steamed. Choose organic food whenever possible. Eat a carrot, eat an apple, have a small salad without dressing, eat an exotic new fruit. The key is to eat a wide variety of colors to ensure you receive a broad spectrum of vitamins, minerals, and nutrients.

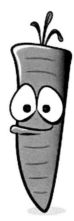

Enjoy the color, aroma, textures, and tastes of eating food in its most beneficial form!

Your body will love you for it!

4. Acknowledge Yourself

If I asked you how many good things
you did today, what would you say?

If I asked you to stand up tall and say
"I am a great and worthwhile person!"
Could you say it with complete integrity
because you really know **you are a great person**?
I hope so, but you'd be surprised how many people can't.

Part of a healthy life involves having a positive self-image. Everyday, we do lots of good things, but we rarely take time to acknowledge what we do. Sometimes we even trivialize our actions as normal or expected. If we can't complete a bazillion tasks in a day, drive a hot car, or live in a fancy home, we might think we are not as good a person as we could be. This kind of attitude leads to the slow tarnishing of our self-image. The lower our self-image gets, the less inclined we become to be our best. **Everything** suffers; our relationships, our health, our families, our work or school, our leisure activities, and our mental abilities. This can grind us down until we actually believe that we *are* insignificant.

The truth of the matter is, you do a multitude of good and worthwhile things each and every day. It's time you start acknowledging yourself for them. Remember, what we focus on expands. The more we put energy, attention, and focus on the good things we do, and the good things in our lives, the more good things will come into our lives.

> *What you believe about you,*
> *impacts you more*
> *than what others believe about you.*
>
> Bill Bartmann

It's time to build a habit of acknowledging the many good things you do. At the end of the day write down at least five good things you did during your day. Here are some examples:
- *I held the door open for a stranger*
- *I gave Susan a sincere compliment just to brighten her day*
- *I told Jack that I appreciate his efforts*
- *I helped with household chores*
- *I completed all my daily tasks in my Healthy Habit Former*
- *I volunteered at the seniors home today*
- *I finally sat down and did my taxes*
- *I took a few moments to sit quietly and admire nature*
- *I sent a card to Mom to let her know I love her*
- *I phoned Janet to apologize*
- *I smiled at a stranger today*

Take time to reflect on your accomplishments as you do this process.

Notice how tremendous you feel!

2.05

Weekly Acceleration Tools:

These four activities will be done once every week

1. *List 5 benefits of exercising regularly*
2. *List 5 ways that anyone can make time for exercise*
3. *Visualize your vibrant, healthy body*
4. *Appreciate your magnificent body*

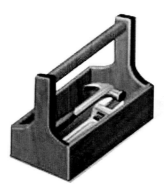

These **once-per-week** activities take only a few minutes to complete. Although these activities may seem simplistic, or a bit unusual, they have extraordinarily powerful consequences that will accelerate your results. Trust the process, do them all, and do them thoroughly, every time.

1. List at least 5 benefits of exercising regularly

Superficially, you *know* that exercise is good for you. Yet, you may not have a habit of exercising consistently.

One method of strengthening your desire to exercise is to periodically take a few minutes to really think about all the benefits exercise can have in your life. So, that is precisely what you are going to do!

> *Your present-day habits will determine which you do later in life -*
> *take two pills or two stairs at a time*
>
> Astrid Whiting

Each week I will ask you to sit down, and list at least five benefits you can derive from regular exercise. For instance:

- *Fat release*
- *Increased overall energy level*
- *Calmer, clearer mind*
- *Strengthened heart*
- *Lower blood pressure*
- *Relieved depression symptoms*
- *Increased muscle tone*
- *Better balance and coordination*
- *Increased bone density*
- *Improved elimination*
- *Elevated mood*
- *Improved self-esteem*
- *Improved circulation*
- *Better quality of life*

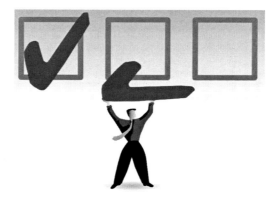

2. List at least 5 ways you can make time for exercise

When is the last time you exercised three times a week consistently? Why did you stop? Did you get busy? Did your life fill up? Was it hard to fit it in?

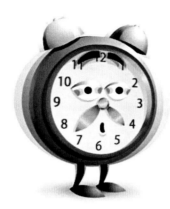

Well, we all live busy lives. Everyday is a full day, and consequently, exercise often gets put on the backburner. Time slips by, and pretty soon you haven't been exercising for a year or more. Then when you're ready to get back to exercise, it suddenly seems hard to find the time.

A busy lifestyle demands strength, and energy. Exercise will condition your body, sharpen your mind, strengthen your muscles, and provide higher levels of energy and stamina. Remember, you've embarked on the *Healthy Habit Former* program to create a healthy, active lifestyle. Part of this process involves ensuring you create time to exercise on a regular basis.

> ### You have all the time that there is.
> Dan Millman

Once a week, I'll ask you to sit down and list five ways that you can make time to exercise. In creating your list, start by examining your current habits and patterns, and decide which of them can be modified or thrown out completely. I want you to find at least five ways you can create thirty minutes, three times a week, to exercise. Here are some examples of what others are doing:

- *Getting up thirty minutes earlier*
- *Cutting out some TV programs*
- *Reading only the newspaper headlines*
- *Letting someone else to do the dishes*
- *Exercising during your lunch break*
- *Allowing someone else to make dinner*
- *Spending thirty minutes less time on the computer*
- *Allowing someone else to do some of the household chores*

2.08

3. Visualization

How fast do you want to create your healthy lifestyle habits? If you're like most people you want to have healthy habits **right now**. I know, that you know, that it takes time to break old habits, and solidly entrench new ones that will last. But, I also know you want it all to happen right now, don't you? I am going to help.

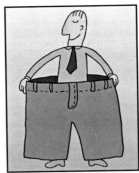

At the beginning of this book, I told you that the *Healthy Habit Former* action plan incorporates strategies to accelerate your results. Using visualization is one of those tools.

Here's how it works. The body cannot tell the difference between what is real, and what is vividly imagined. Numerous studies have shown that when athletes **visualize** specific moves, their muscles react as if that action was really happening.

> *All that we are*
> *is the result of what we have thought.*
>
> Buddha

The point I want to make here is that vivid visualization, combined with practicing your other healthy habits, will accelerate your results.

At least once a week I want you to take a few minutes to sit back, close your eyes, and visualize the ideal healthier you. This is a relaxing, and enjoyable process. Many people find they like to do this daily. The key to this process is to incorporate as much detail as you can. Make your vision as vivid as possible.
- *Examine in detail what every part of your body looks like*
- *Notice how you feel*
- *See yourself doing all the things you can now do in a vibrant body*

The more vivid and specific your visualization, the more your mind will engage your body to make your vision a reality.

To learn more about this incredibly powerful process I invite you to visit our website at www.SynergenixFitness.com . Once there, go the *Achieve Your Vibrant Healthy Body* page, and listen to: *The Power of Visualization* a 10min interview with bestselling author, and clinical hypnotherapist, Dr. Brian Walsh. If you really want to accelerate your results, purchase my self-hypnosis guided visualization CD *Achieve Your Vibrant Healthy Body*. It's an ideal companion for the *Healthy Habit Former* program.

4. Appreciate Your Magnificent Body

Too often we forget just how amazing our body really is. We get caught up in spending all our time thinking about what we *want to be,* and dismiss what we already are.

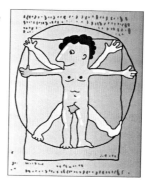

Quantum physics proves that when we show appreciation for anyone or anything, magic happens. Your body, and mind are connected. Because of this connection changes actually occur at the cellular level in your body when you convey an attitude of appreciation.

When you put this principle of quantum physics to practice you will accelerate your results in becoming a vibrant, healthy person. The more you acknowledge just how magnificent your body is right now, the more your body will physically change to become even healthier. Additionally, having gratitude for what you already have will encourage you to make healthy choices more regularly.

> ### When we change the way we look at things, the things we look at change.
>
> Anonymous

Begin a habit of being grateful for your magnificent body. Once a week, I want you to list at least three things you appreciate about your body right now. For instance:

- *Having a strong heart*
- *Being free of disease*
- *Ability to think clearly*
- *Having a good memory*
- *The ability to simply walk*
- *Being able to see, speak, and /or hear*
- *Having a digestive system that works well*
- *Having two arms, and two legs*
- *Being able to breathe freely*

Next, describe *why* you are grateful, and how that makes you *feel.* The more vivid your description the better. For example:

> *I am so grateful that I have two working legs. I can walk, run and just generally be mobile. Being this mobile affords me great freedoms in life. I can independently go where I want anytime without having to rely on anyone. I have the option to strengthen my legs to increase my mobility, agility, stability, and balance so that I can even begin to participate in activities that demand a little more. How fortunate I am to have that option. I am very grateful for this because I know there are many people in the world who have lost the use of their legs or don't even have legs. I feel truly grateful for my ability to simply walk. Wow, what a gift.*

> ### You do not need to know how things work; You need to know that they work.
>
> Anonymous

Healthy Habit Former

Exercise Days: Exercise 3 times each week

Could you stand to release a little fat? Would you like a stronger heart? How about a stronger more efficient body? Would you enjoy a sense of overall physical and mental wellbeing? Yes? Okay, then you need to exercise regularly.

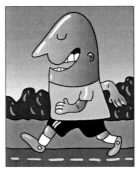

By the time you get to this point in your program, you will have already been thinking about the benefits of exercise, and ways to make time for exercise. *Now it's time to actually exercise.*

In the *Healthy Habit Former*, you will focus on aerobic/cardio (cardiovascular) exercise. This type of exercise can strengthen the heart, improve circulation, improve breathing, promote fat release, lower blood pressure, lessen or eliminate Type 2 Diabetes, improve balance and stability, increase overall strength, improve mental clarity, and release endorphins – the bodies 'feel good' drug.

One important note about exercise is to be sure that you enjoy yourself when doing it. Often, when people begin an exercise program they go too fast or too hard, they do an activity they don't like, put themselves in environment they don't like, then end up feeling uncomfortable, unhappy, then quit. That is not the way to entrench the exercise habit. I know this seems a little silly, but you'd be surprised how many people believe that exercise has to be uncomfortable, or even hurt, to be beneficial. That's just plain BOGUS! **Exercise should always feel good!**

> *A bear, however hard he tries,*
> *grows tubby without exercise.*
>
> Winnie the Pooh

The key to exercise adherence is to exercise at a pace that is right for YOU. Do the activity that is right for YOU. Exercise in surroundings that feel good to YOU. When you feel comfortable exercising, and you enjoy what you are doing, you are much more likely to make exercise a habit!

2.11

To begin your habit of regular exercise, commit to aerobic exercise three times a week, for at least 30 minutes each time. *Make sure you have obtained your doctor's approval before beginning.*

Make your 30 minutes of exercise **continuous and enjoyable**. Once you start moving, keep moving for the entire 30 minutes. No stopping and starting, keep going. Speed is not really important.

Proper warm up and cool down periods *are* important during cardiovascular exercise. You can incorporate these easily by following this simple "pace pattern" during your 30 minutes of exercise:

5 minutes slow pace - 20 minutes faster pace - 5 minutes slow

People often wonder what *speed* constitutes slow, medium or fast. Whatever speed *feels* slow, medium or fast *to you* is accurate.

Here are some examples of aerobic/cardio exercise you can do:

- ♥ Walking
- ♥ Swimming lengths
- ♥ Biking outside
- ♥ Ice Skating
- ♥ Nordic Walking
- ♥ Stationary cycling
- ♥ Any "Aerobic" type class
- ♥ Treadmill walking or jogging

- ♥ Jogging/running
- ♥ Hiking
- ♥ Cross-country skiing
- ♥ Rollerblading
- ♥ Stair-climbing machine
- ♥ Elliptical Training
- ♥ Freewheel class
- ♥ Aquafit class

Healthy Habit Former

Days 30, 60, and 90

When you make incremental improvements on a daily basis, you don't always realize just how much you have accomplished over time. Taking time to look backward at where you were is vital to acknowledging how far you have come. If you don't do this from time to time you might trivialize your accomplishments, or feel that you aren't really progressing at all. This is especially true when creating new habits, because this process is gradual.

An integral part of the *Healthy Habit Former* program is for you to periodically pause to measure your progress.

> *Today's mighty oak is simply yesterday's nut that held it's ground.*
>
> Anonymous

So, on Day 30, 60, and 90 I want you to perform two tasks:
1. Reflect on your progress
2. Celebrate your successes

First. I will assist you in reflecting on your progress by asking you to flip through the pages of your action plan, and then respond to some specific questions. This will be a fun, and your results may surprise you.

2.13

Next, you get to celebrate!

That's right. You get to celebrate.
Whoop it up a bit!

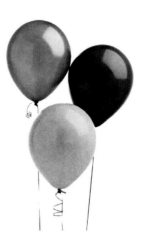

After all, by day 30, 60 and 90 you have been diligent in creating healthy habits. You absolutely deserve to celebrate!

Celebrating your success sends a strong message to the subconscious. The subconscious learns that living healthy is rewarded in a positive way. Since the body, mind, and spirit like to be rewarded, the subconscious will keep sending messages to your conscious mind to reinforce the positive behaviors that brought you to this day to celebrate.

Celebrate in any way you like. The key to celebrating, is to **do something out of the ordinary,** so the subconscious takes note of it. It doesn't have to be huge or expensive, just different. Here are some examples of ways you can celebrate:

- *Have a special dinner*
- *Buy some flowers*
- *Take a day off to do anything you want*
- *Go to a movie*
- *Get a massage*
- *Sleep in*
- *Have breakfast in bed*
- *Enjoy a special beverage*
- *Enjoy a quiet evening at home alone*
- *Sit in a hot tub or take a long quiet bath*
- *Go to the theatre*
- *Listen to some live music*
- *Go to the beach and relax*
- *Rent a canoe*
- *Go fishing*

Whatever you do, be creative, and have fun.

> *The more you praise and celebrate your life,*
> *the more there is in life to celebrate.*
>
> Oprah Winfrey

Sample Daily Sheet

So far we have covered why, and how to perform each of the activities in your *Healthy Habit Former* action plan. To summarize, you'll start each day by opening up your action plan, filling in the date, and completing the first activity. Then, simply read the remaining activities, incorporate them into your day, and log what you have done. Here's a sample of what one of your daily sheets might look like.

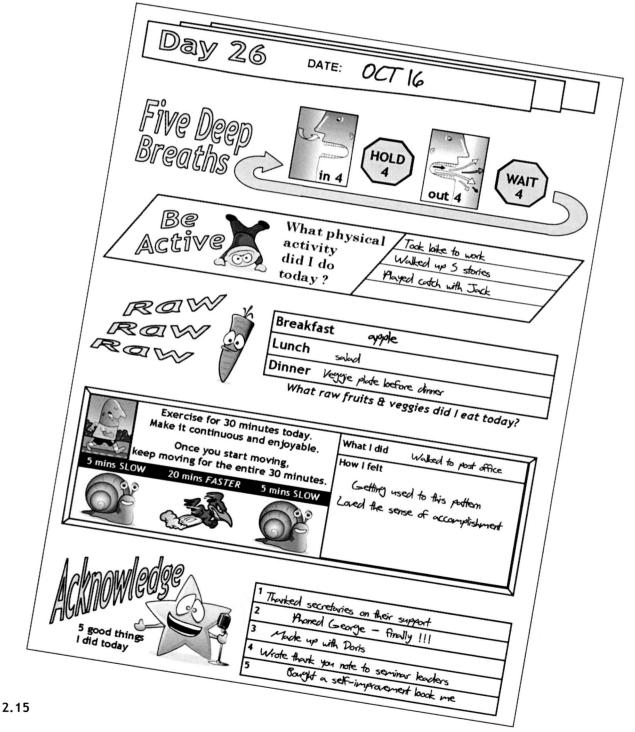

Getting the Most out of Your Experience

Following the **Healthy Habit Former** program day-by-day, step-by-step will absolutely create healthy, active lifestyle habits. You will discover new and fascinating things about yourself and your body.

Make your **Healthy Habit Former** program an enjoyable experience. Approach each new day with a sense of openness and curiosity. Be adventurous in choosing a new raw food, exercise in beautiful and comfortable surroundings, work at your own pace, and enjoy your few minutes of peace and quiet when you just simply breathe.

The more you make the process enjoyable, the easier and faster you will create healthier lifestyle habits. Be kind to yourself. Work at your own pace. Be comfortable. If you miss a day or two, not to worry, re-start where you left off. Just keep going.

Now, are you ready?
Let's create some healthy, active lifestyle habits...

> *Take care of your body.*
> *It's the only place you have to live.*
>
> Jim Rohn

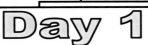 **Day 1** DATE:

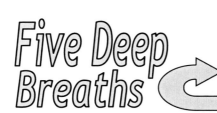 **Five Deep Breaths** 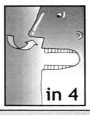 in 4 HOLD 4 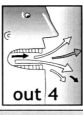 out 4 WAIT 4

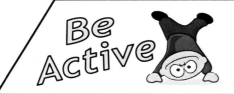 **Be Active**

What physical activity did I do today ?

Raw Raw Raw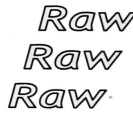

Breakfast	
Lunch	
Dinner	

What raw fruits & veggies did I eat today?

List five benefits of exercising regularly

1	
2	
3	
4	
5	

Acknowledge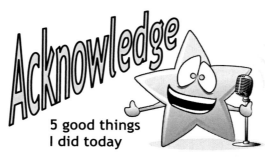

5 good things I did today

1	
2	
3	
4	
5	

Day 2

DATE:

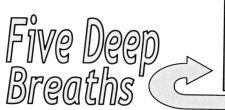 **Five Deep Breaths**

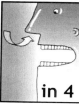 in 4   HOLD 4 out 4 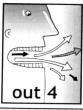 WAIT 4

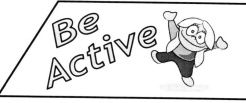 **Be Active**

What physical activity did I do today?

Raw Raw Raw

Breakfast	
Lunch	
Dinner	

What raw fruits & veggies did I eat today?

List five ways that anyone can make time for exercise

1	
2	
3	
4	
5	

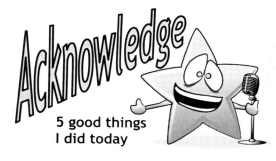 **Acknowledge**

5 good things I did today

1	
2	
3	
4	
5	

Healthy Habit Former

Day 3

DATE:

Five Deep Breaths

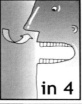 in 4 **HOLD 4** out 4 **WAIT 4**

Be Active

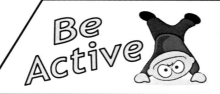

What physical activity did I do today ?

Raw Raw Raw

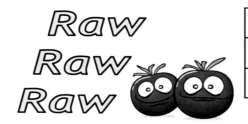

Breakfast
Lunch
Dinner

What raw fruits & veggies did I eat today?

Exercise at least 30 minutes today.
Make it continuous and enjoyable.

Once you start moving,
keep moving for the entire time.

What I did
How I felt

5 mins SLOW   **20 mins *FASTER***   **5 mins SLOW**

 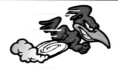

Acknowledge

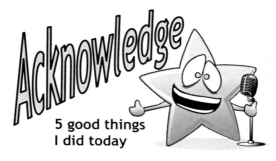

5 good things
I did today

1
2
3
4
5

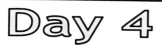

Day 4   DATE:

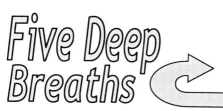

Five Deep Breaths

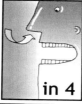
in 4

HOLD 4

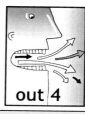
out 4

WAIT 4

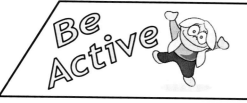

Be Active

What physical activity did I do today ?

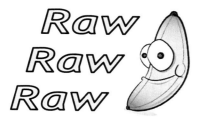

Raw Raw Raw

| Breakfast |
| Lunch |
| Dinner |

What raw fruits & veggies did I eat today?

Take a minute, close your eyes, visualize the ideal healthier you.
What do you look like?   What can you do?   How do you feel?

Describe your vision

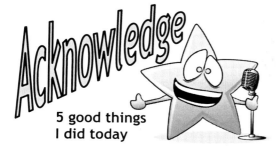

Acknowledge

5 good things I did today

| 1 |
| 2 |
| 3 |
| 4 |
| 5 |

Day 5   DATE:

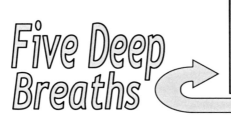Five Deep Breaths

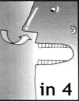 in 4   HOLD 4   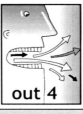 out 4   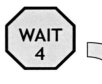WAIT 4

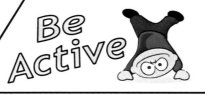Be Active

What physical activity did I do today ?

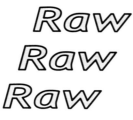Raw Raw Raw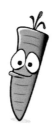

| Breakfast |
| Lunch |
| Dinner |

What raw fruits & veggies did I eat today?

Exercise at least 30 minutes today.
Make it continuous and enjoyable.

Once you start moving,
keep moving for the entire time.

| What I did |
| How I felt |

| 5 mins SLOW | 20 mins *FASTER* | 5 mins SLOW |

 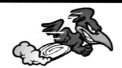

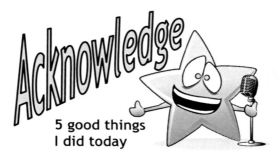Acknowledge

5 good things
I did today

1	
2	
3	
4	
5	

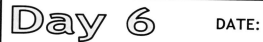

Day 6   DATE:

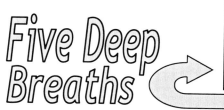 Five Deep Breaths

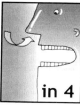 in 4

HOLD 4

 out 4

WAIT 4

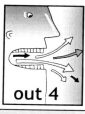

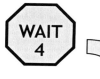

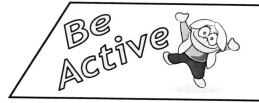 Be Active

What physical activity did I do today?

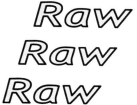 Raw Raw Raw

Breakfast
Lunch
Dinner

What raw fruits & veggies did I eat today?

Appreciate Your Magnificent Body
List at least three things you appreciate about your body right now.

1   2   3

Pick one, and describe why you're grateful How do you feel about that?

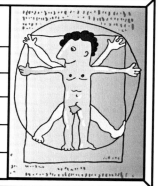

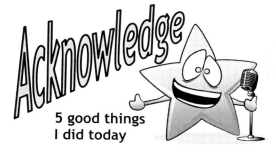 Acknowledge

5 good things I did today

1
2
3
4
5

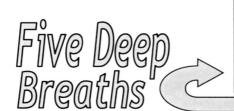

Five Deep Breaths

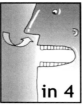 in 4   HOLD 4   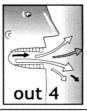 out 4   WAIT 4

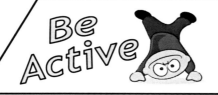

Be Active

What physical activity did I do today ?

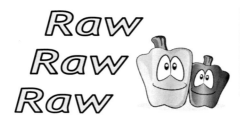

Raw Raw Raw

| Breakfast |
| Lunch |
| Dinner |

What raw fruits & veggies did I eat today?

Exercise at least 30 minutes today. Make it continuous and enjoyable.

Once you start moving, keep moving for the entire time.

| 5 mins SLOW | 20 mins *FASTER* | 5 mins SLOW |

What I did

How I felt

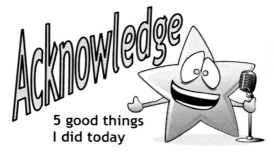

Acknowledge

5 good things I did today

| 1 |
| 2 |
| 3 |
| 4 |
| 5 |

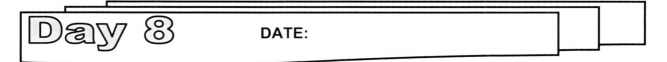

Day 8

DATE:

Five Deep Breaths

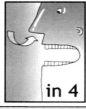 in 4   HOLD 4 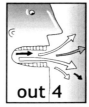 out 4   WAIT 4

Be Active

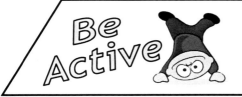

What physical activity did I do today?

Raw Raw Raw

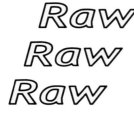

| Breakfast |
| Lunch |
| Dinner |

What raw fruits & veggies did I eat today?

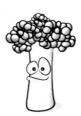

List five benefits of exercising regularly

| 1 |
| 2 |
| 3 |
| 4 |
| 5 |

Acknowledge

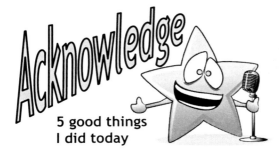

5 good things I did today

| 1 |
| 2 |
| 3 |
| 4 |
| 5 |

Day 9

DATE:

Five Deep Breaths

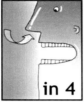 in 4

 HOLD 4

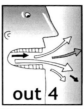 out 4

 WAIT 4

Be Active

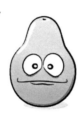

What physical activity did I do today?

Raw Raw Raw

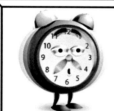

Breakfast
Lunch
Dinner

What raw fruits & veggies did I eat today?

List five ways that anyone can make time for exercise

1	
2	
3	
4	
5	

Acknowledge

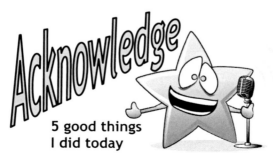

5 good things I did today

1	
2	
3	
4	
5	

Day 10   DATE:

Five Deep Breaths

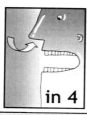 in 4   HOLD 4   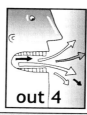 out 4   WAIT 4

Be Active
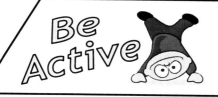

What physical activity did I do today?

Raw Raw Raw
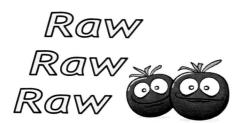

Breakfast	
Lunch	
Dinner	

What raw fruits & veggies did I eat today?

 Exercise at least 30 minutes today. Make it continuous and enjoyable.

Once you start moving, keep moving for the entire time.

| 5 mins SLOW | 20 mins *FASTER* | 5 mins SLOW |

 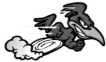

What I did

How I felt

Acknowledge

5 good things I did today

1	
2	
3	
4	
5	

Day 11

DATE:

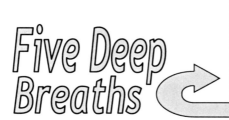

Five Deep Breaths

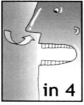 in 4

 HOLD 4

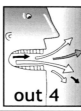 out 4

 WAIT 4

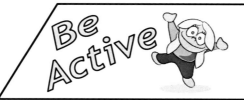

Be Active

What physical activity did I do today?

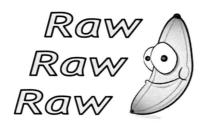

Raw Raw Raw

Breakfast	
Lunch	
Dinner	

What raw fruits & veggies did I eat today?

Take a minute, close your eyes, visualize the ideal healthier you.
What do you look like?   What can you do?   How do you feel?

Describe your vision

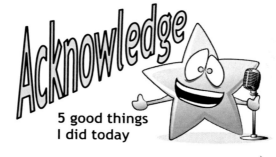

Acknowledge

5 good things I did today

1	
2	
3	
4	
5	

Day 12   DATE:

Five Deep Breaths

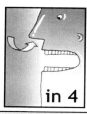 in 4   HOLD 4   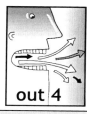 out 4   WAIT 4

Be Active

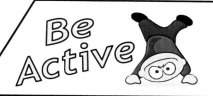

What physical activity did I do today?

Raw Raw Raw

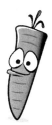

Breakfast	
Lunch	
Dinner	

What raw fruits & veggies did I eat today?

 Exercise at least 30 minutes today. Make it continuous and enjoyable.

Once you start moving, keep moving for the entire time.

5 mins SLOW	20 mins *FASTER*	5 mins SLOW
	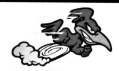	

What I did

How I felt

Acknowledge

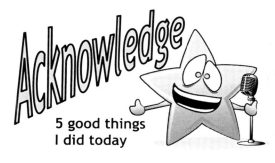

5 good things I did today

1	
2	
3	
4	
5	

Day 13

DATE:

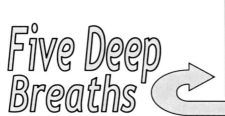

Five Deep Breaths

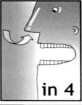 in 4

 HOLD 4

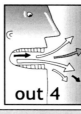 out 4

 WAIT 4

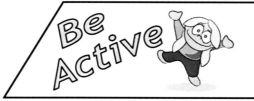

Be Active

What physical activity did I do today?

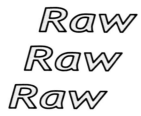

Raw Raw Raw

Breakfast	
Lunch	
Dinner	

What raw fruits & veggies did I eat today?

Appreciate Your Magnificent Body
List at least three things you appreciate about your body right now.

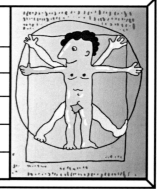

1	2	3

Pick one, and describe why you're grateful How do you feel about that?

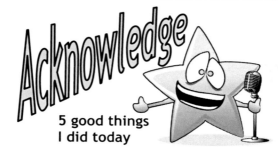

Acknowledge

5 good things I did today

1	
2	
3	
4	
5	

Day 14   DATE:

Five Deep Breaths

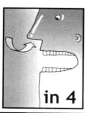 in 4   HOLD 4   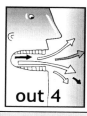 out 4   WAIT 4

Be Active

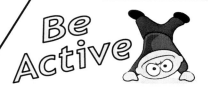

What physical activity did I do today ?

Raw Raw Raw

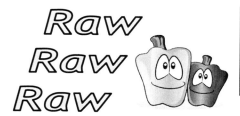

Breakfast	
Lunch	
Dinner	

What raw fruits & veggies did I eat today?

Exercise at least 30 minutes today.
Make it continuous and enjoyable.

Once you start moving,
keep moving for the entire time.

What I did	
How I felt	

5 mins SLOW	20 mins *FASTER*	5 mins SLOW

 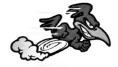

Acknowledge

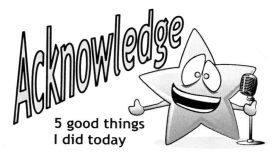

5 good things
I did today

1	
2	
3	
4	
5	

Day 15

DATE:

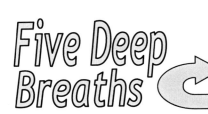

Five Deep Breaths

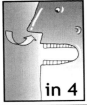 in 4   HOLD 4   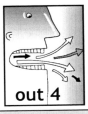 out 4   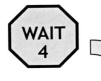 WAIT 4

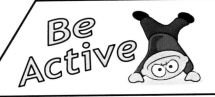

Be Active

What physical activity did I do today?

Raw Raw Raw

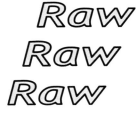

Breakfast	
Lunch	
Dinner	

What raw fruits & veggies did I eat today?

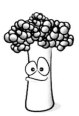

List five benefits of exercising regularly

1	
2	
3	
4	
5	

Acknowledge

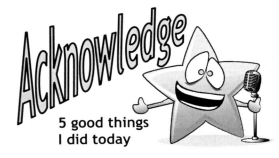

5 good things I did today

1	
2	
3	
4	
5	

Day 16   DATE:

Five Deep Breaths

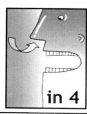 in 4   HOLD 4   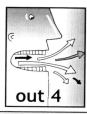 out 4   WAIT 4

Be Active

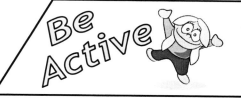

What physical activity did I do today ?

Raw Raw Raw

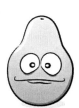

Breakfast	
Lunch	
Dinner	

What raw fruits & veggies did I eat today?

List five ways that anyone can make time for exercise

1	
2	
3	
4	
5	

Acknowledge

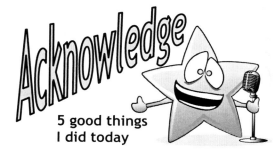

5 good things I did today

1	
2	
3	
4	
5	

Day 17

DATE:

Five Deep Breaths

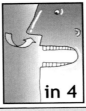 **in 4** **HOLD 4**   **out 4** **WAIT 4**

Be Active

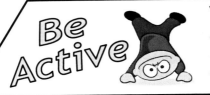

What physical activity did I do today ?

Raw Raw Raw

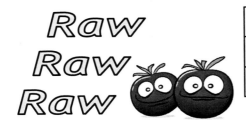

Breakfast
Lunch
Dinner

What raw fruits & veggies did I eat today?

 Exercise at least 30 minutes today.
Make it continuous and enjoyable.

Once you start moving,
keep moving for the entire time.

5 mins SLOW	20 mins *FASTER*	5 mins SLOW

 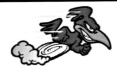

What I did
How I felt

Acknowledge

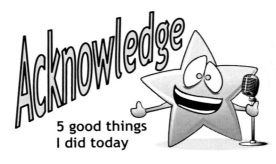

**5 good things
I did today**

1	
2	
3	
4	
5	

Day 18

DATE:

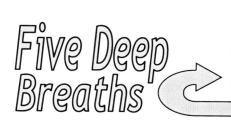 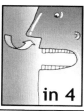 HOLD 4 in 4 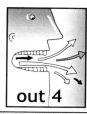 WAIT 4 out 4

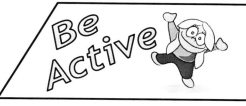 **What physical activity did I do today ?**

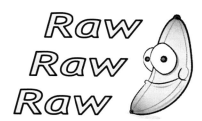

Breakfast	
Lunch	
Dinner	

What raw fruits & veggies did I eat today?

Take a minute, close your eyes, visualize the ideal healthier you.
What do you look like?   What can you do?   How do you feel?

Describe your vision

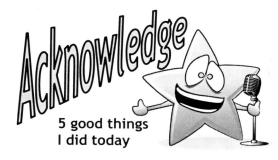

5 good things I did today

1	
2	
3	
4	
5	

Day 19

DATE:

Five Deep Breaths

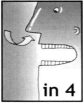 in 4   HOLD 4 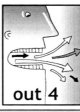 out 4   WAIT 4

Be Active

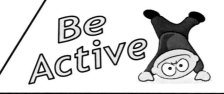

What physical activity did I do today?

Raw Raw Raw

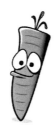

Breakfast
Lunch
Dinner

What raw fruits & veggies did I eat today?

Exercise at least 30 minutes today. Make it continuous and enjoyable.

Once you start moving, keep moving for the entire time.

What I did
How I felt

5 mins SLOW **20 mins *FASTER*** **5 mins SLOW**

 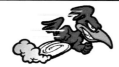

Acknowledge

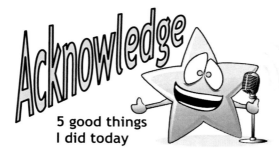

5 good things I did today

1
2
3
4
5

Day 20   DATE:

Five Deep Breaths

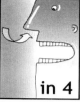 in 4   HOLD 4   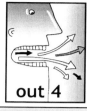 out 4   WAIT 4

Be Active

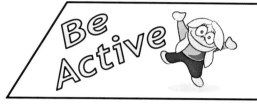

What physical activity did I do today?

Raw Raw Raw

Breakfast	
Lunch	
Dinner	

What raw fruits & veggies did I eat today?

Appreciate Your Magnificent Body

List at least three things you appreciate about your body right now.

1	2	3

Pick one, and describe why you're grateful How do you feel about that?

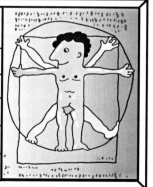

Acknowledge

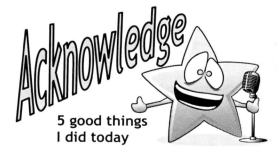

5 good things I did today

1	
2	
3	
4	
5	

Day 21

DATE:

Five Deep Breaths

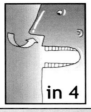 in 4 HOLD 4 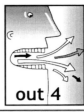 out 4 WAIT 4

Be Active

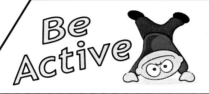

What physical activity did I do today ?

Raw Raw Raw

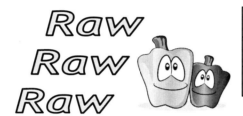

Breakfast	
Lunch	
Dinner	

What raw fruits & veggies did I eat today?

Exercise at least 30 minutes today. Make it continuous and enjoyable.

Once you start moving, keep moving for the entire time.

5 mins SLOW   20 mins *FASTER*   5 mins SLOW

What I did
How I felt

Acknowledge

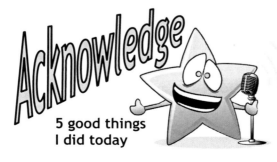

5 good things I did today

1	
2	
3	
4	
5	

Day 22

DATE:

Five Deep Breaths

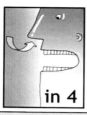 in 4   HOLD 4 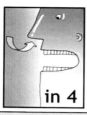 out 4   WAIT 4

Be Active

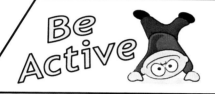

What physical activity did I do today ?

Raw Raw Raw

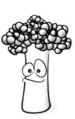

Breakfast
Lunch
Dinner

What raw fruits & veggies did I eat today?

List five benefits of exercising regularly

1	
2	
3	
4	
5	

Acknowledge

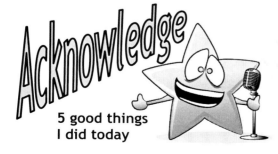

5 good things I did today

1	
2	
3	
4	
5	

Day 23   DATE:

Five Deep Breaths

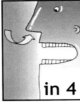 in 4   HOLD 4   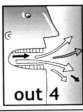 out 4   WAIT 4

Be Active

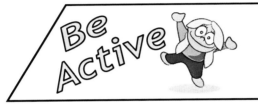

What physical activity did I do today?

Raw Raw Raw

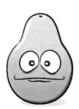

Breakfast	
Lunch	
Dinner	

What raw fruits & veggies did I eat today?

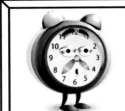

List five ways that anyone can make time for exercise

1	
2	
3	
4	
5	

Acknowledge

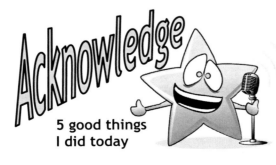

5 good things I did today

1	
2	
3	
4	
5	

Day 24

DATE:

Five Deep Breaths

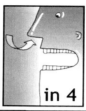 in 4   HOLD 4   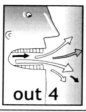 out 4   WAIT 4

Be Active

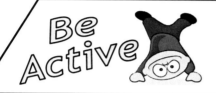

What physical activity did I do today ?

Raw Raw Raw

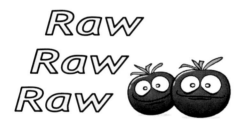

| Breakfast |
| Lunch |
| Dinner |

What raw fruits & veggies did I eat today?

Exercise at least 30 minutes today.
Make it continuous and enjoyable.

Once you start moving,
keep moving for the entire time.

5 mins SLOW   20 mins *FASTER*   5 mins SLOW

| What I did |
| How I felt |

Acknowledge

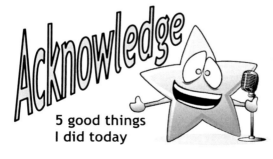

5 good things
I did today

1	
2	
3	
4	
5	

Day 25

DATE:

Five Deep Breaths

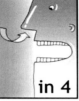 in 4 HOLD 4 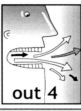 out 4 WAIT 4

Be Active

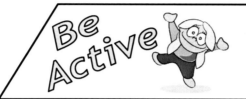

What physical activity did I do today ?

Raw Raw Raw

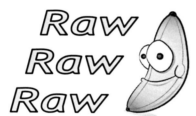

Breakfast
Lunch
Dinner

What raw fruits & veggies did I eat today?

Take a minute, close your eyes, visualize the ideal healthier you.
What do you look like?   What can you do?   How do you feel?

Describe your vision

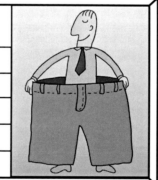

Acknowledge

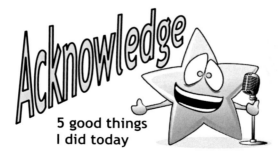

5 good things I did today

1
2
3
4
5

Day 26

DATE:

Five Deep Breaths

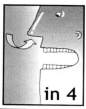 in 4 HOLD 4 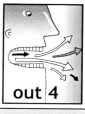 out 4 WAIT 4

Be Active

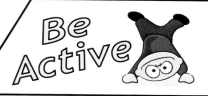

What physical activity did I do today ?

Raw Raw Raw

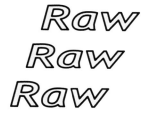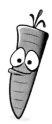

Breakfast	
Lunch	
Dinner	

What raw fruits & veggies did I eat today?

Exercise at least 30 minutes today. Make it continuous and enjoyable. Once you start moving, keep moving for the entire time.	What I did
	How I felt

5 mins SLOW	20 mins *FASTER*	5 mins SLOW

 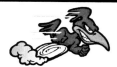

Acknowledge

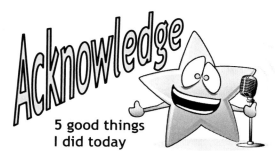

5 good things I did today

1	
2	
3	
4	
5	

Day 27

DATE:

Five Deep Breaths

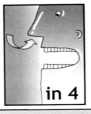 in 4

 HOLD 4

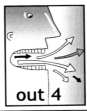 out 4

 WAIT 4

Be Active

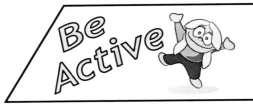

What physical activity did I do today ?

Raw Raw Raw

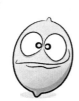

| Breakfast |
| Lunch |
| Dinner |

What raw fruits & veggies did I eat today?

Appreciate Your Magnificent Body

List at least three things you appreciate about your body right now.

| 1 | 2 | 3 |

Pick one, and describe why you're grateful How do you feel about that?

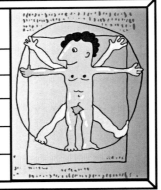

Acknowledge

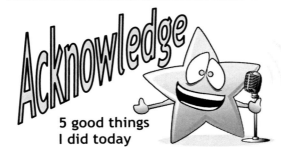

5 good things I did today

| 1 |
| 2 |
| 3 |
| 4 |
| 5 |

Day 28

DATE:

Five Deep Breaths

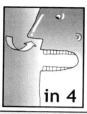 in 4   HOLD 4 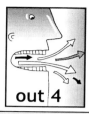 out 4   WAIT 4

Be Active

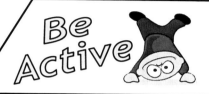

What physical activity did I do today?

Raw Raw Raw

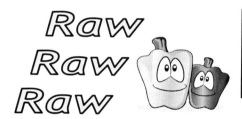

Breakfast
Lunch
Dinner

What raw fruits & veggies did I eat today?

Exercise at least 30 minutes today.
Make it continuous and enjoyable.

Once you start moving,
keep moving for the entire time.

5 mins SLOW	20 mins *FASTER*	5 mins SLOW

 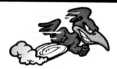

What I did
How I felt

Acknowledge

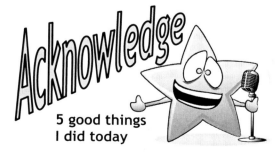

5 good things I did today

1	
2	
3	
4	
5	

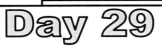 **Day 29**   DATE:

Five Deep Breaths 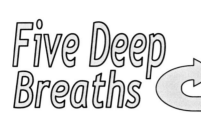 in 4 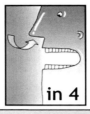 HOLD 4 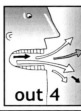 out 4 WAIT 4

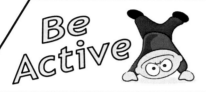 **Be Active**   What physical activity did I do today ?

Raw Raw Raw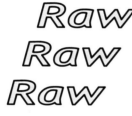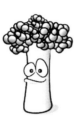

| Breakfast |
| Lunch |
| Dinner |

What raw fruits & veggies did I eat today?

List five benefits of exercising regularly

1
2
3
4
5

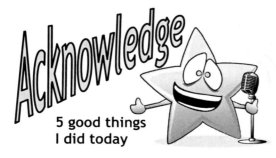 **Acknowledge**

5 good things I did today

1
2
3
4
5

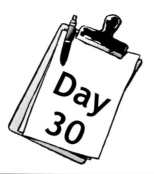

Day 30

Date

Reflect on your Progress

*Take a few minutes to flip back
through the pages of the last thirty days.*

Over the last 30 days, what activities were the most fun,
and easiest to incorporate in to your life?
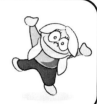

What new fruits or vegetables did you experience over the last 30 days?
What value are you receiving from eating raw foods?
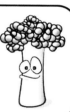

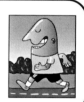
What benefits have you noticed from exercising regularly?
What are you enjoying most about your exercise routine?

What have you learned about yourself over the last 30 days?

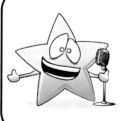

Congratulations..

You've just reached a milestone.
It's time to give yourself a pat on the back, and celebrate this achievement.

Get out there and treat yourself to something special. You deserve it.

Day 31

DATE:

Five Deep Breaths

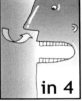 in 4 HOLD 4 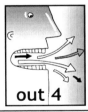 out 4 WAIT 4

Be Active

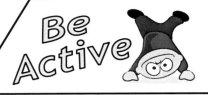

What physical activity did I do today ?

Raw Raw Raw

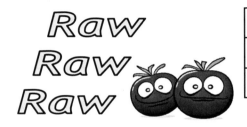

Breakfast
Lunch
Dinner

What raw fruits & veggies did I eat today?

 Exercise at least 30 minutes today. Make it continuous and enjoyable.

Once you start moving, keep moving for the entire time.

5 mins SLOW   **20 mins *FASTER***   **5 mins SLOW**

 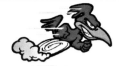

What I did
How I felt

Acknowledge

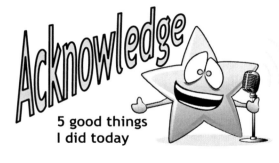

5 good things I did today

1	
2	
3	
4	
5	

Day 32

DATE:

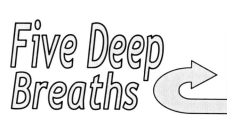 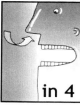 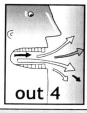

in 4   HOLD 4   out 4   WAIT 4

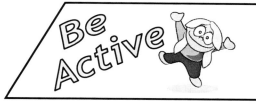

What physical activity did I do today ?

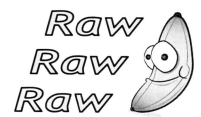

| Breakfast |
| Lunch |
| Dinner |

What raw fruits & veggies did I eat today?

Take a minute, close your eyes, visualize the ideal healthier you.
What do you look like?   What can you do?   How do you feel?

Describe your vision

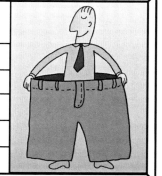

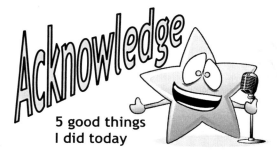

5 good things I did today

| 1 |
| 2 |
| 3 |
| 4 |
| 5 |

Day 33 — DATE:

Five Deep Breaths

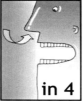 in 4   HOLD 4   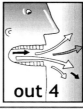 out 4   WAIT 4

Be Active

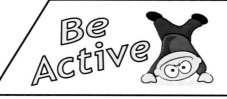

What physical activity did I do today ?

Raw Raw Raw

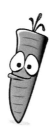

| Breakfast |
| Lunch |
| Dinner |

What raw fruits & veggies did I eat today?

Exercise at least 30 minutes today. Make it continuous and enjoyable.

Once you start moving, keep moving for the entire time.

| 5 mins SLOW | 20 mins *FASTER* | 5 mins SLOW |

 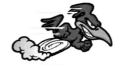

| What I did |
| How I felt |

Acknowledge

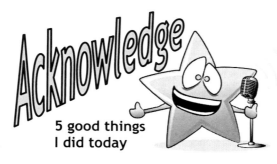

5 good things I did today

| 1 |
| 2 |
| 3 |
| 4 |
| 5 |

Day 34

DATE:

Five Deep Breaths

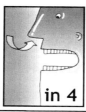 in 4   HOLD 4   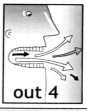 out 4   WAIT 4

Be Active

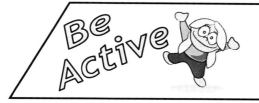

What physical activity did I do today ?

Raw Raw Raw

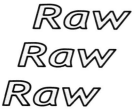

| Breakfast |
| Lunch |
| Dinner |

What raw fruits & veggies did I eat today?

Appreciate Your Magnificent Body

List at least three things you appreciate about your body right now.

| 1 | 2 | 3 |

Pick one, and describe why you're grateful How do you feel about that?

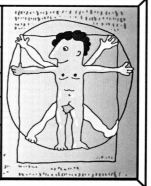

Acknowledge

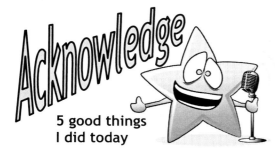

5 good things I did today

| 1 |
| 2 |
| 3 |
| 4 |
| 5 |

Day 35   DATE:

Five Deep Breaths

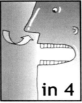 in 4   HOLD 4   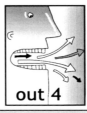 out 4   WAIT 4

Be Active

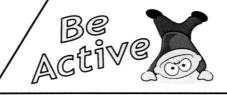

What physical activity did I do today?

Raw Raw Raw

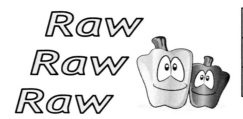

Breakfast	
Lunch	
Dinner	

What raw fruits & veggies did I eat today?

 Exercise at least 30 minutes today. Make it continuous and enjoyable.

Once you start moving, keep moving for the entire time.

5 mins SLOW	20 mins *FASTER*	5 mins SLOW
	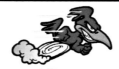	

What I did
How I felt

Acknowledge

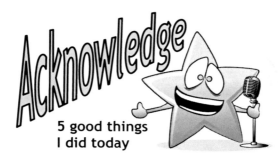

5 good things I did today

1	
2	
3	
4	
5	

Day 36

DATE:

Five Deep Breaths

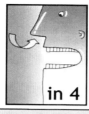 in 4   HOLD 4   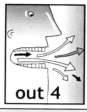 out 4   WAIT 4

Be Active

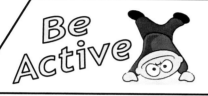

What physical activity did I do today ?

Raw Raw Raw

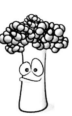

| Breakfast |
| Lunch |
| Dinner |

What raw fruits & veggies did I eat today?

List five benefits of exercising regularly

1
2
3
4
5

Acknowledge

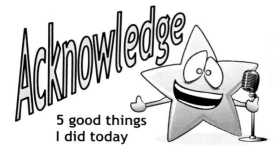

5 good things I did today

1
2
3
4
5

Day 37

DATE: _____

Five Deep Breaths

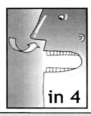 in 4 HOLD 4 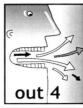 out 4 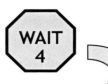 WAIT 4

Be Active

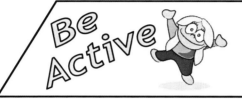

What physical activity did I do today?

_____
_____
_____

Raw Raw Raw

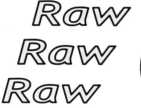

Breakfast	
Lunch	
Dinner	

What raw fruits & veggies did I eat today?

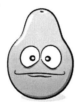

List five ways that anyone can make time for exercise

1 _____
2 _____
3 _____
4 _____
5 _____

Acknowledge

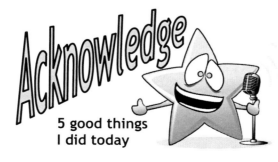

5 good things I did today

1 _____
2 _____
3 _____
4 _____
5 _____

Five Deep Breaths

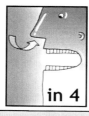 **in 4**   **HOLD 4** 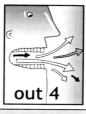 **out 4**   **WAIT 4**

Be Active

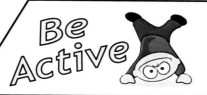

What physical activity did I do today ?

Raw Raw Raw

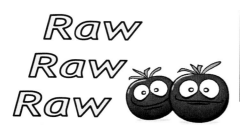

| Breakfast |
| Lunch |
| Dinner |

What raw fruits & veggies did I eat today?

Exercise at least 30 minutes today. Make it continuous and enjoyable.

Once you start moving, keep moving for the entire time.

5 mins SLOW   20 mins *FASTER*   5 mins SLOW

What I did

How I felt

Acknowledge

5 good things I did today

| 1 |
| 2 |
| 3 |
| 4 |
| 5 |

Day 39

DATE:

Five Deep Breaths

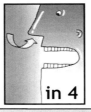 in 4 HOLD 4 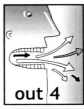 out 4 WAIT 4

Be Active

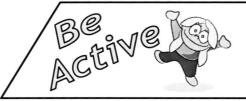

What physical activity did I do today ?

Raw Raw Raw

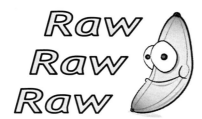

| Breakfast |
| Lunch |
| Dinner |

What raw fruits & veggies did I eat today?

Take a minute, close your eyes, visualize the ideal healthier you.
What do you look like?   What can you do?   How do you feel?

Describe your vision

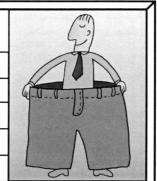

Acknowledge

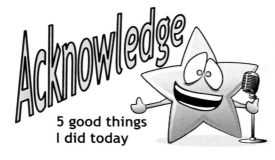

5 good things I did today

| 1 |
| 2 |
| 3 |
| 4 |
| 5 |

Day 40

DATE:

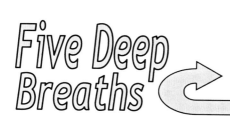

Five Deep Breaths

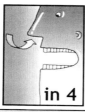 in 4   **HOLD 4**   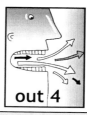 out 4   **WAIT 4**

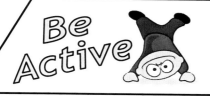 **Be Active**

What physical activity did I do today?

Raw Raw Raw

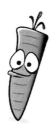

| Breakfast |
| Lunch |
| Dinner |

What raw fruits & veggies did I eat today?

Exercise at least 30 minutes today. Make it continuous and enjoyable.

Once you start moving, keep moving for the entire time.

| 5 mins SLOW | 20 mins *FASTER* | 5 mins SLOW |

 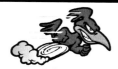

What I did

How I felt

Acknowledge

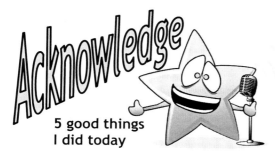

5 good things I did today

| 1 |
| 2 |
| 3 |
| 4 |
| 5 |

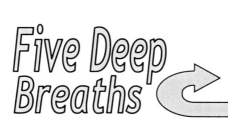

Five Deep Breaths

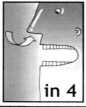

in 4

HOLD 4

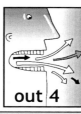

out 4

WAIT 4

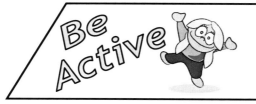

Be Active

What physical activity did I do today?

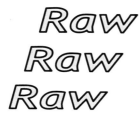

Raw Raw Raw

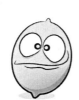

| Breakfast |
| Lunch |
| Dinner |

What raw fruits & veggies did I eat today?

Appreciate Your Magnificent Body

List at least three things you appreciate about your body right now.

1   2   3

Pick one, and describe why you're grateful How do you feel about that?

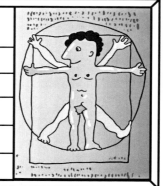

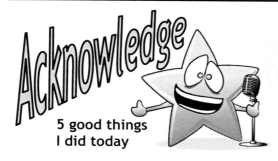

Acknowledge

5 good things I did today

| 1 |
| 2 |
| 3 |
| 4 |
| 5 |

Day 42

DATE:

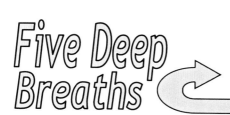

Five Deep Breaths

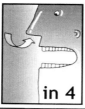 in 4   HOLD 4   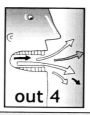 out 4   WAIT 4

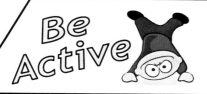

Be Active

What physical activity did I do today ?

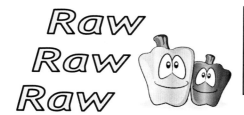

Raw Raw Raw

Breakfast	
Lunch	
Dinner	

What raw fruits & veggies did I eat today?

Exercise at least 30 minutes today.
Make it continuous and enjoyable.

Once you start moving,
keep moving for the entire time.

5 mins SLOW	20 mins *FASTER*	5 mins SLOW

 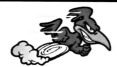

What I did	
How I felt	

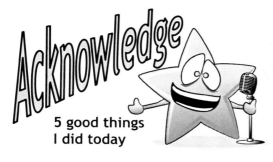

Acknowledge

5 good things I did today

1	
2	
3	
4	
5	

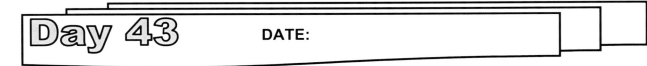

Day 43

DATE:

Five Deep Breaths

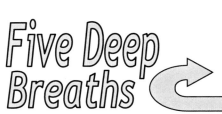
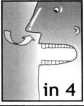

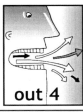

in 4   HOLD 4   out 4   WAIT 4

Be Active

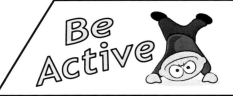

What physical activity did I do today ?

Raw Raw Raw

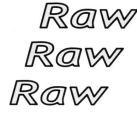

Breakfast	
Lunch	
Dinner	

What raw fruits & veggies did I eat today?

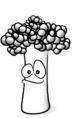

List five benefits of exercising regularly

1	
2	
3	
4	
5	

Acknowledge

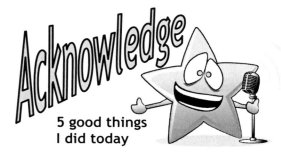

5 good things I did today

1	
2	
3	
4	
5	

Day 44   DATE:

Five Deep Breaths

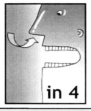 in 4   HOLD 4   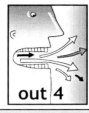 out 4   WAIT 4

Be Active

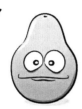

What physical activity did I do today ?

Raw Raw Raw

Breakfast	
Lunch	
Dinner	

What raw fruits & veggies did I eat today?

List five ways that anyone can make time for exercise

1	
2	
3	
4	
5	

Acknowledge

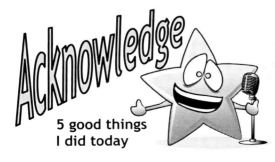

5 good things I did today

1	
2	
3	
4	
5	

Day 45　　DATE:

Five Deep Breaths

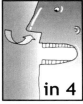 in 4　 HOLD 4　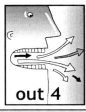 out 4　 WAIT 4

Be Active

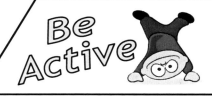

What physical activity did I do today ?

Raw Raw Raw

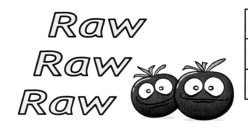

Breakfast	
Lunch	
Dinner	

What raw fruits & veggies did I eat today?

 Exercise at least 30 minutes today.
Make it continuous and enjoyable.

Once you start moving,
keep moving for the entire time.

5 mins SLOW　20 mins *FASTER*　5 mins SLOW

 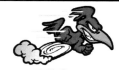

What I did	
How I felt	

Acknowledge

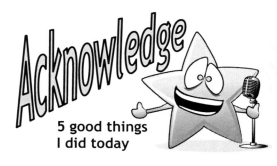

5 good things
I did today

1	
2	
3	
4	
5	

Day 46

DATE:

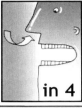 in 4

HOLD 4

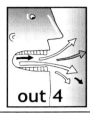 out 4

WAIT 4

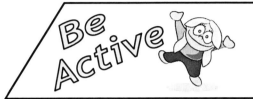

What physical activity did I do today?

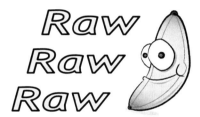

Breakfast	
Lunch	
Dinner	

What raw fruits & veggies did I eat today?

Take a minute, close your eyes, visualize the ideal healthier you.
What do you look like?   What can you do?   How do you feel?

Describe your vision

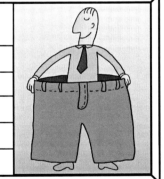

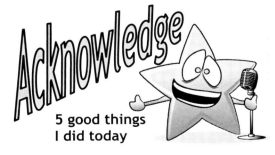

5 good things I did today

1	
2	
3	
4	
5	

©2007 Synergenix Fitness   *Healthy Habit Former*   www.SynergenixFitness.com

Day 47   DATE:

Five Deep Breaths

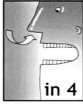 in 4   HOLD 4   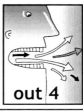 out 4   WAIT 4

Be Active

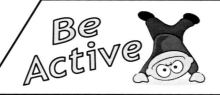

What physical activity did I do today?

Raw Raw Raw

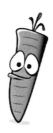

Breakfast	
Lunch	
Dinner	

What raw fruits & veggies did I eat today?

Exercise at least 30 minutes today. Make it continuous and enjoyable.

Once you start moving, keep moving for the entire time.

What I did	
How I felt	

5 mins SLOW   20 mins *FASTER*   5 mins SLOW

 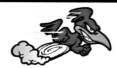

Acknowledge

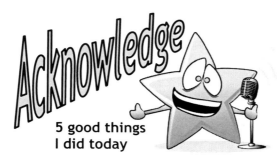

5 good things I did today

1	
2	
3	
4	
5	

Healthy Habit Former

Day 48

DATE:

Five Deep Breaths

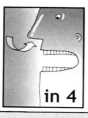 in 4   HOLD 4   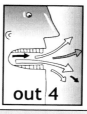 out 4   WAIT 4

Be Active

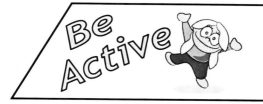

What physical activity did I do today ?

Raw Raw Raw

Breakfast
Lunch
Dinner

What raw fruits & veggies did I eat today?

Appreciate Your Magnificent Body

List at least three things you appreciate about your body right now.

1	2	3

Pick one, and describe why you're grateful How do you feel about that?

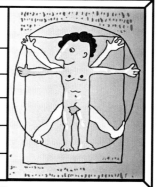

Acknowledge

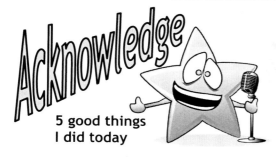

5 good things I did today

1	
2	
3	
4	
5	

Day 49

DATE:

Five Deep Breaths

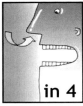 in 4   HOLD 4 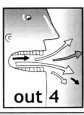 out 4   WAIT 4

Be Active

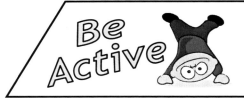

What physical activity did I do today ?

Raw Raw Raw

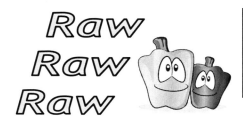

Breakfast	
Lunch	
Dinner	

What raw fruits & veggies did I eat today?

Exercise at least 30 minutes today.
Make it continuous and enjoyable.

Once you start moving,
keep moving for the entire time.

| 5 mins SLOW | 20 mins *FASTER* | 5 mins SLOW |

 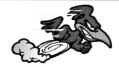

What I did

How I felt

Acknowledge

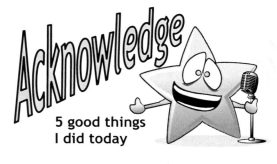

5 good things
I did today

1	
2	
3	
4	
5	

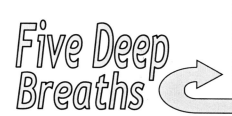

Day 50

DATE:

Five Deep Breaths

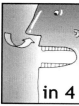 in 4

 HOLD 4

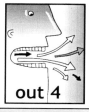 out 4

 WAIT 4

Be Active

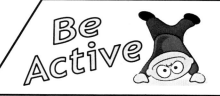

What physical activity did I do today ?

Raw Raw Raw

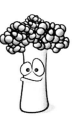

Breakfast	
Lunch	
Dinner	

What raw fruits & veggies did I eat today?

1	
2	
3	
4	
5	

List five benefits of exercising regularly

Acknowledge

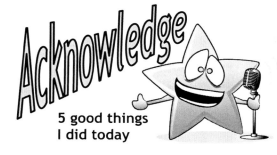

5 good things I did today

1	
2	
3	
4	
5	

Day 51   DATE:

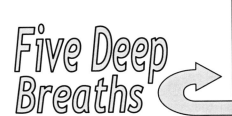 Five Deep Breaths 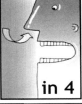 in 4   HOLD 4   out 4   WAIT 4

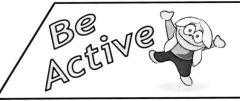 Be Active   What physical activity did I do today ?

Raw Raw Raw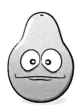

Breakfast	
Lunch	
Dinner	

What raw fruits & veggies did I eat today?

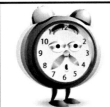

List five ways that anyone can make time for exercise

1	
2	
3	
4	
5	

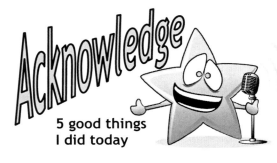 Acknowledge

5 good things I did today

1	
2	
3	
4	
5	

Day 52   DATE:

Five Deep Breaths

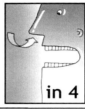 in 4   HOLD 4   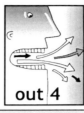 out 4   WAIT 4

Be Active

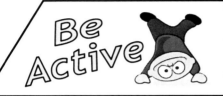 What physical activity did I do today ?

Raw Raw Raw

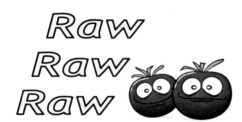

Breakfast	
Lunch	
Dinner	

What raw fruits & veggies did I eat today?

Exercise at least 30 minutes today.
Make it continuous and enjoyable.

Once you start moving,
keep moving for the entire time.

5 mins SLOW	20 mins *FASTER*	5 mins SLOW
	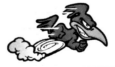	

What I did
How I felt

Acknowledge

5 good things I did today

1	
2	
3	
4	
5	

Day 53   DATE:

Five Deep Breaths

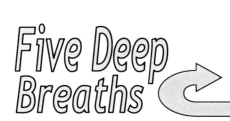 **in 4**   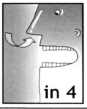 **HOLD 4**   **out 4**   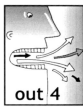 **WAIT 4**

Be Active

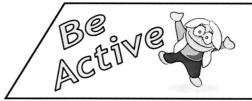

What physical activity did I do today ?

Raw Raw Raw

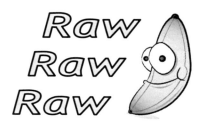

Breakfast	
Lunch	
Dinner	

What raw fruits & veggies did I eat today?

Take a minute, close your eyes, visualize the ideal healthier you.
What do you look like?   What can you do?   How do you feel?

Describe your vision

Acknowledge

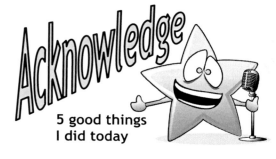

5 good things I did today

1	
2	
3	
4	
5	

Day 54

DATE:

Five Deep Breaths

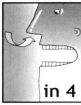 in 4

 HOLD 4

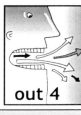 out 4

 WAIT 4

Be Active

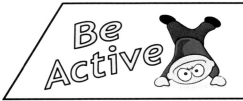

What physical activity did I do today?

Raw Raw Raw

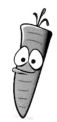

Breakfast	
Lunch	
Dinner	

What raw fruits & veggies did I eat today?

Exercise at least 30 minutes today.
Make it continuous and enjoyable.

Once you start moving,
keep moving for the entire time.

5 mins SLOW	20 mins *FASTER*	5 mins SLOW

 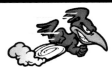

What I did

How I felt

Acknowledge

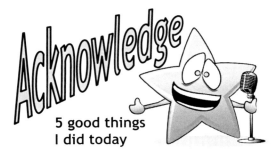

5 good things I did today

1	
2	
3	
4	
5	

Day 55   DATE:

Five Deep Breaths

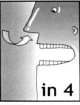 in 4   HOLD 4   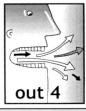 out 4   WAIT 4

Be Active

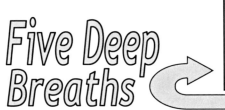

What physical activity did I do today ?

Raw Raw Raw

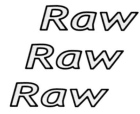

Breakfast	
Lunch	
Dinner	

What raw fruits & veggies did I eat today?

Appreciate Your Magnificent Body
List at least three things you appreciate about your body right now.

1	2	3

Pick one, and describe why you're grateful How do you feel about that?

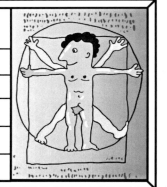

Acknowledge

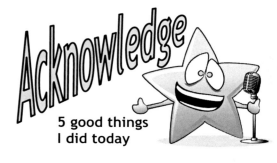

5 good things I did today

1	
2	
3	
4	
5	

Day 56

DATE:

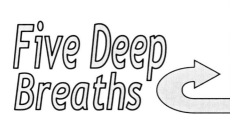

Five Deep Breaths

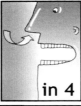 in 4

 HOLD 4

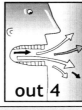 out 4

 WAIT 4

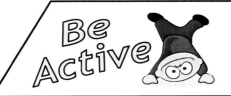

Be Active

What physical activity did I do today?

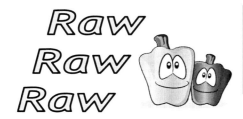

Raw Raw Raw

Breakfast	
Lunch	
Dinner	

What raw fruits & veggies did I eat today?

Exercise at least 30 minutes today.
Make it continuous and enjoyable.

Once you start moving,
keep moving for the entire time.

5 mins SLOW 20 mins *FASTER* 5 mins SLOW

  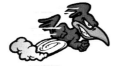

What I did	
How I felt	

Acknowledge

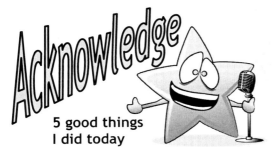

5 good things I did today

1	
2	
3	
4	
5	

Day 57

DATE:

Five Deep Breaths

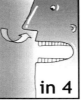 in 4   HOLD 4   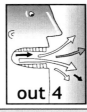 out 4   WAIT 4

Be Active

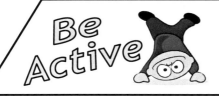

What physical activity did I do today ?

Raw Raw Raw

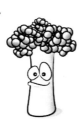

Breakfast	
Lunch	
Dinner	

What raw fruits & veggies did I eat today?

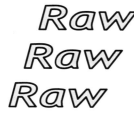

List five benefits of exercising regularly

1	
2	
3	
4	
5	

Acknowledge

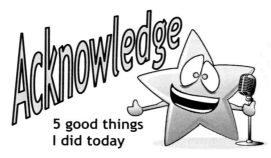

5 good things I did today

1	
2	
3	
4	
5	

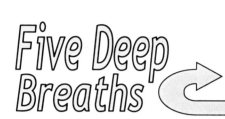 **Five Deep Breaths**

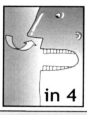 in 4   HOLD 4   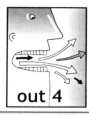 out 4   WAIT 4

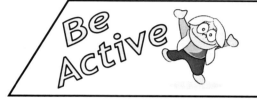 **Be Active**   What physical activity did I do today ?

Raw Raw Raw

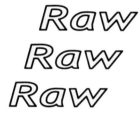

Breakfast	
Lunch	
Dinner	

What raw fruits & veggies did I eat today?

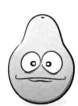

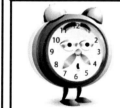

List five ways that anyone can make time for exercise

1	
2	
3	
4	
5	

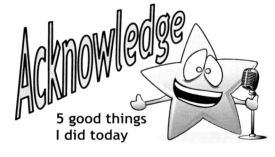 **Acknowledge**

5 good things I did today

1	
2	
3	
4	
5	

Day 59

DATE:

Five Deep Breaths

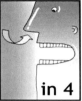 in 4   **HOLD 4** 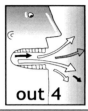 out 4   **WAIT 4**

Be Active

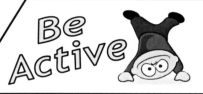

What physical activity did I do today?

Raw Raw Raw

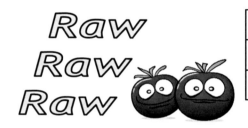

Breakfast	
Lunch	
Dinner	

What raw fruits & veggies did I eat today?

Exercise at least 30 minutes today.
Make it continuous and enjoyable.

Once you start moving,
keep moving for the entire time.

What I did	
How I felt	

 5 mins SLOW   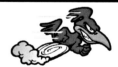 **20 mins *FASTER***   **5 mins SLOW**

Acknowledge

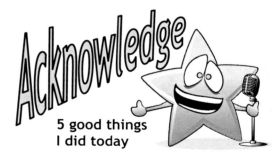

5 good things
I did today

1	
2	
3	
4	
5	

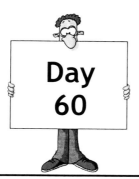

Day 60

Reflect on your Progress

Take a few minutes to flip back
through the pages of the last thirty days.

Over the last 30 days, what activities were the most fun,
and easiest to incorporate in to your life?

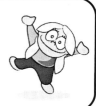

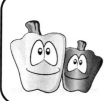

What new fruits or vegetables did you experience over the last 30 days?
What value are you receiving from eating raw foods?

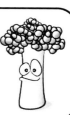

What benefits have you noticed from exercising regularly?
What are you enjoying most about your exercise routine?

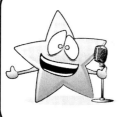

What have you learned about yourself over the last 30 days?

Way to go...

You're two-thirds of the way there!
It's time to celebrate this achievement.

Remember, make it something fun and extraordinary.

Have a fantastic day!

Day 61   DATE:

Five Deep Breaths

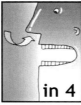 in 4   HOLD 4   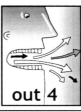 out 4   WAIT 4

Be Active

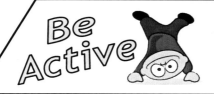

What physical activity did I do today ?

Raw Raw Raw

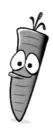

Breakfast	
Lunch	
Dinner	

What raw fruits & veggies did I eat today?

 Exercise at least 30 minutes today.
Make it continuous and enjoyable.

Once you start moving,
keep moving for the entire time.

5 mins SLOW	20 mins *FASTER*	5 mins SLOW

 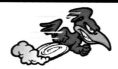

What I did	
How I felt	

Acknowledge

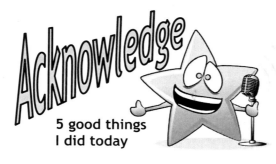

**5 good things
I did today**

1	
2	
3	
4	
5	

Five Deep Breaths

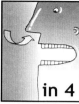 in 4   HOLD 4   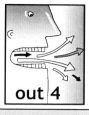 out 4   WAIT 4

Be Active

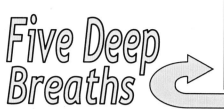 What physical activity did I do today ?

Raw Raw Raw

| Breakfast |
| Lunch |
| Dinner |

What raw fruits & veggies did I eat today?

Appreciate Your Magnificent Body

List at least three things you appreciate about your body right now.

1   2   3

Pick one, and describe why you're grateful How do you feel about that?

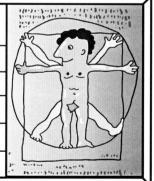

Acknowledge

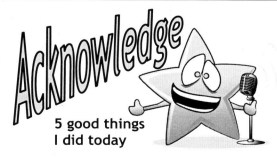

5 good things I did today

| 1 |
| 2 |
| 3 |
| 4 |
| 5 |

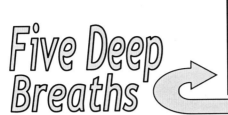

Five Deep Breaths

 in 4
 HOLD 4
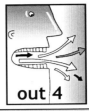 out 4
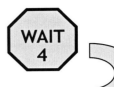 WAIT 4

Be Active

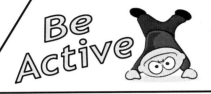

What physical activity did I do today ?

Raw Raw Raw

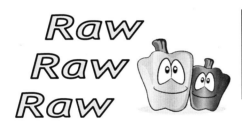

Breakfast	
Lunch	
Dinner	

What raw fruits & veggies did I eat today?

 Exercise at least 30 minutes today. Make it continuous and enjoyable.

Once you start moving, keep moving for the entire time.

What I did	
How I felt	

5 mins SLOW   20 mins *FASTER*   5 mins SLOW

 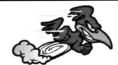

Acknowledge

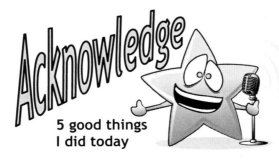

5 good things I did today

1	
2	
3	
4	
5	

Day 64

DATE:

Five Deep Breaths

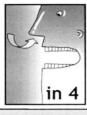 in 4   HOLD 4   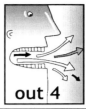 out 4   WAIT 4

Be Active

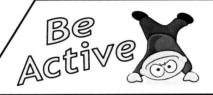

What physical activity did I do today ?

Raw Raw Raw

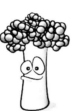

Breakfast	
Lunch	
Dinner	

What raw fruits & veggies did I eat today?

List five benefits of exercising regularly

1	
2	
3	
4	
5	

Acknowledge

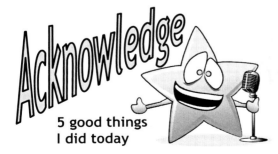

5 good things I did today

1	
2	
3	
4	
5	

Day 65

DATE:

Five Deep Breaths

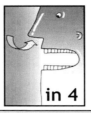 in 4 HOLD 4 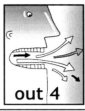 out 4 WAIT 4

Be Active

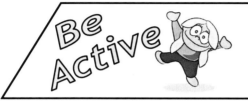

What physical activity did I do today?

Raw Raw Raw

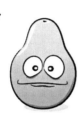

Breakfast	
Lunch	
Dinner	

What raw fruits & veggies did I eat today?

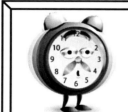

List five ways that anyone can make time for exercise

1	
2	
3	
4	
5	

Acknowledge

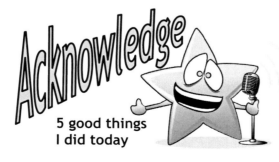

5 good things I did today

1	
2	
3	
4	
5	

Day 66

DATE:

Five Deep Breaths

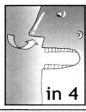 in 4   HOLD 4   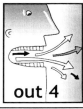 out 4   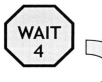 WAIT 4

Be Active

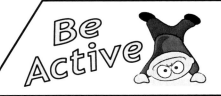

What physical activity did I do today?

Raw Raw Raw

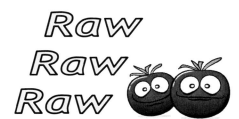

Breakfast
Lunch
Dinner

What raw fruits & veggies did I eat today?

Exercise at least 30 minutes today.
Make it continuous and enjoyable.

Once you start moving,
keep moving for the entire time.

What I did
How I felt

5 mins SLOW   20 mins *FASTER*   5 mins SLOW

   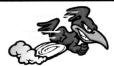

Acknowledge

5 good things
I did today

1	
2	
3	
4	
5	

Day 67

DATE:

Five Deep Breaths

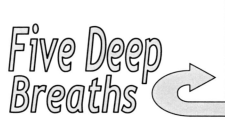

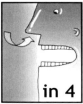 in 4   HOLD 4 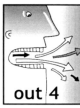 out 4   WAIT 4

Be Active

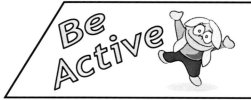

What physical activity did I do today?

Raw Raw Raw

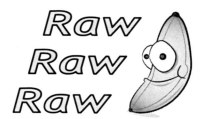

Breakfast
Lunch
Dinner

What raw fruits & veggies did I eat today?

Take a minute, close your eyes, visualize the ideal healthier you.
What do you look like?   What can you do?   How do you feel?

Describe your vision

Acknowledge

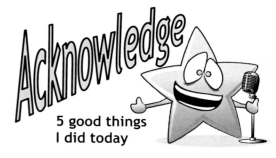

5 good things I did today

1
2
3
4
5

Day 68

DATE:

Five Deep Breaths

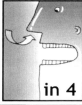 in 4 HOLD 4 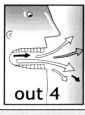 out 4 WAIT 4

Be Active

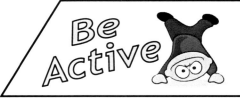

What physical activity did I do today?

Raw Raw Raw

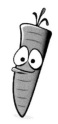

Breakfast	
Lunch	
Dinner	

What raw fruits & veggies did I eat today?

Exercise at least 30 minutes today.
Make it continuous and enjoyable.

Once you start moving,
keep moving for the entire time.

| 5 mins SLOW | 20 mins *FASTER* | 5 mins SLOW |

 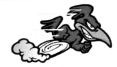

| What I did | |
| How I felt | |

Acknowledge

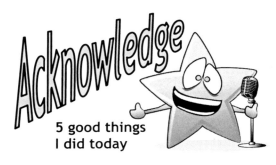

5 good things
I did today

1	
2	
3	
4	
5	

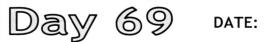

Day 69   DATE:

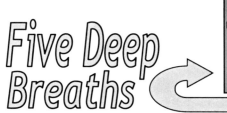

Five Deep Breaths

 in 4   HOLD 4   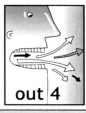 out 4   WAIT 4

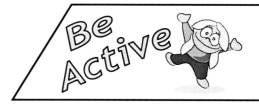

Be Active

What physical activity did I do today?

Raw Raw Raw

Breakfast
Lunch
Dinner

What raw fruits & veggies did I eat today?

Appreciate Your Magnificent Body
List at least three things you appreciate about your body right now.

1	2	3

Pick one, and describe why you're grateful How do you feel about that?

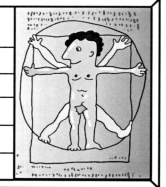

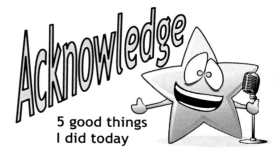

Acknowledge

5 good things
I did today

1
2
3
4
5

Day 70

DATE:

Five Deep Breaths

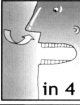 in 4   HOLD 4 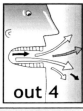 out 4   WAIT 4

Be Active

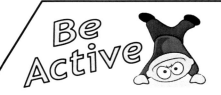

What physical activity did I do today ?

Raw Raw Raw

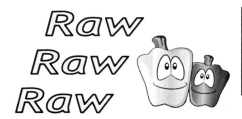

| Breakfast |
| Lunch |
| Dinner |

What raw fruits & veggies did I eat today?

Exercise at least 30 minutes today.
Make it continuous and enjoyable.

Once you start moving,
keep moving for the entire time.

| 5 mins SLOW | 20 mins *FASTER* | 5 mins SLOW |

 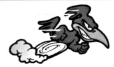

What I did

How I felt

Acknowledge

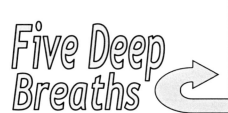

5 good things
I did today

1	
2	
3	
4	
5	

Day 71

DATE:

Five Deep Breaths

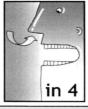 in 4
 HOLD 4
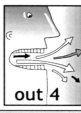 out 4
 WAIT 4

Be Active

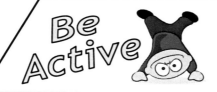

What physical activity did I do today?

Raw Raw Raw

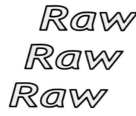

Breakfast
Lunch
Dinner

What raw fruits & veggies did I eat today?

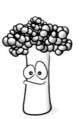

List five benefits of exercising regularly

1	
2	
3	
4	
5	

Acknowledge

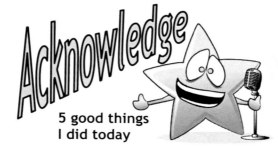

5 good things I did today

1	
2	
3	
4	
5	

Day 72

DATE:

Five Deep Breaths

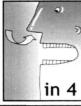 **in 4**
 HOLD 4
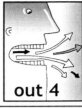 **out 4**
 WAIT 4

Be Active

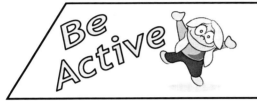

What physical activity did I do today ?

Raw Raw Raw

Breakfast	
Lunch	
Dinner	

What raw fruits & veggies did I eat today?

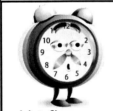

List five ways that anyone can make time for exercise

1	
2	
3	
4	
5	

Acknowledge

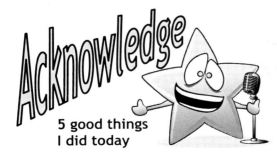

5 good things I did today

1	
2	
3	
4	
5	

Day 73

DATE:

Five Deep Breaths

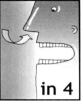 in 4 HOLD 4 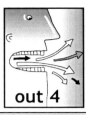 out 4 WAIT 4

Be Active

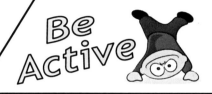

What physical activity did I do today?

Raw Raw Raw

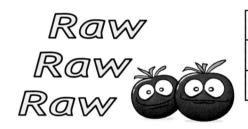

Breakfast	
Lunch	
Dinner	

What raw fruits & veggies did I eat today?

Exercise at least 30 minutes today.
Make it continuous and enjoyable.

Once you start moving,
keep moving for the entire time.

5 mins SLOW	20 mins *FASTER*	5 mins SLOW

 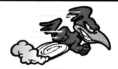

What I did
How I felt

Acknowledge

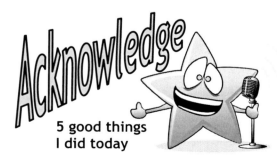

5 good things
I did today

1	
2	
3	
4	
5	

Five Deep Breaths

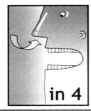 in 4   HOLD 4   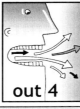 out 4   WAIT 4

Be Active

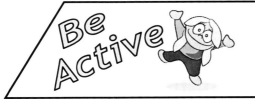

What physical activity did I do today?

Raw Raw Raw

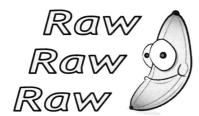

Breakfast	
Lunch	
Dinner	

What raw fruits & veggies did I eat today?

Take a minute, close your eyes, visualize the ideal healthier you.
What do you look like?   What can you do?   How do you feel?

Describe your vision

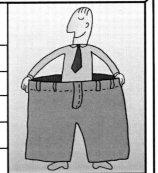

Acknowledge

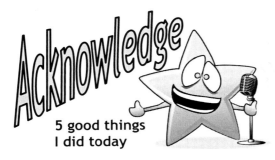

5 good things
I did today

1	
2	
3	
4	
5	

Day 75

DATE:

Five Deep Breaths

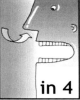 in 4 | HOLD 4 | out 4 | WAIT 4

Be Active

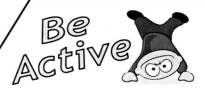

What physical activity did I do today ?

Raw Raw Raw

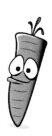

| Breakfast |
| Lunch |
| Dinner |

What raw fruits & veggies did I eat today?

Exercise at least 30 minutes today. Make it continuous and enjoyable.

Once you start moving, keep moving for the entire time.

5 mins SLOW | 20 mins *FASTER* | 5 mins SLOW

 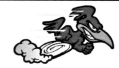

What I did

How I felt

Acknowledge

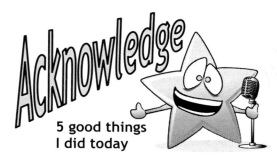

5 good things I did today

| 1 |
| 2 |
| 3 |
| 4 |
| 5 |

Day 76

DATE:

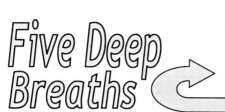 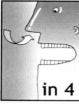 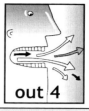

in 4 | HOLD 4 | out 4 | WAIT 4

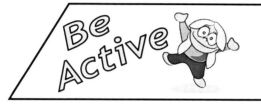

What physical activity did I do today ?

Raw Raw Raw

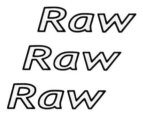

Breakfast
Lunch
Dinner

What raw fruits & veggies did I eat today?

Appreciate Your Magnificent Body
List at least three things you appreciate about your body right now.

1	2	3

Pick one, and describe why you're grateful How do you feel about that?

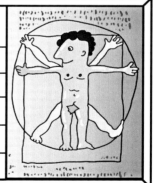

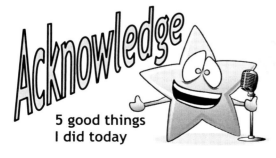

5 good things I did today

1
2
3
4
5

Day 77

DATE:

Five Deep Breaths

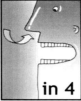 in 4   HOLD 4   out 4 WAIT 4

Be Active

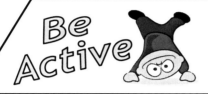 What physical activity did I do today ?

Raw Raw Raw

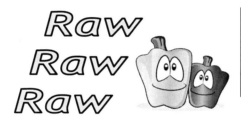

Breakfast	
Lunch	
Dinner	

What raw fruits & veggies did I eat today?

 Exercise at least 30 minutes today.
Make it continuous and enjoyable.

Once you start moving,
keep moving for the entire time.

5 mins SLOW	20 mins *FASTER*	5 mins SLOW

 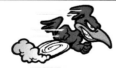

What I did

How I felt

Acknowledge

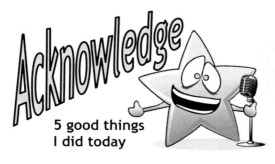

5 good things I did today

1	
2	
3	
4	
5	

Day 78

DATE:

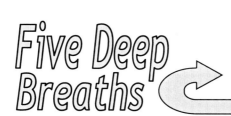

Five Deep Breaths

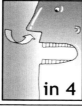 in 4   HOLD 4 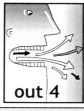 out 4   WAIT 4

Be Active

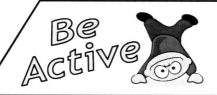

What physical activity did I do today ?

Raw Raw Raw

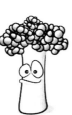

Breakfast	
Lunch	
Dinner	

What raw fruits & veggies did I eat today?

List five benefits of exercising regularly

1	
2	
3	
4	
5	

Acknowledge

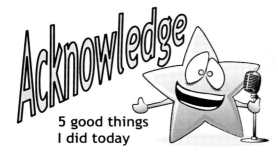

5 good things I did today

1	
2	
3	
4	
5	

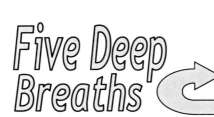

Five Deep Breaths

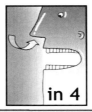 in 4
 HOLD 4
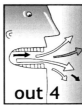 out 4
 WAIT 4

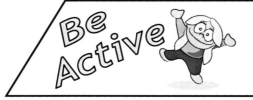

Be Active

What physical activity did I do today ?

Raw Raw Raw

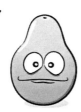

Breakfast
Lunch
Dinner

What raw fruits & veggies did I eat today?

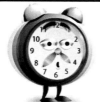

List five ways that anyone can make time for exercise

1	
2	
3	
4	
5	

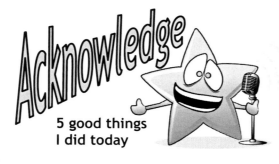

Acknowledge

5 good things I did today

1	
2	
3	
4	
5	

Day 80

DATE:

Five Deep Breaths

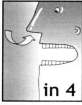 in 4 **HOLD 4** 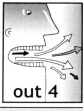 out 4 **WAIT 4**

Be Active

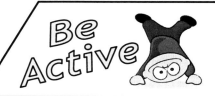

What physical activity did I do today ?

Raw Raw Raw

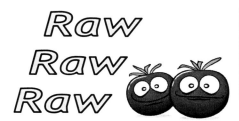

Breakfast	
Lunch	
Dinner	

What raw fruits & veggies did I eat today?

Exercise at least 30 minutes today.
Make it continuous and enjoyable.

Once you start moving,
keep moving for the entire time.

5 mins SLOW	20 mins *FASTER*	5 mins SLOW

 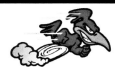

What I did	
How I felt	

Acknowledge

5 good things I did today

1	
2	
3	
4	
5	

Day 81

DATE:

Five Deep Breaths

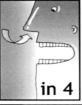 in 4   HOLD 4   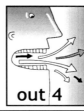 out 4   WAIT 4

Be Active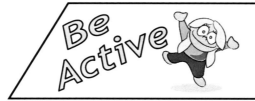

What physical activity did I do today ?

Raw Raw Raw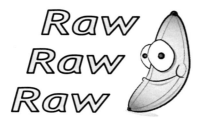

| Breakfast |
| Lunch |
| Dinner |

What raw fruits & veggies did I eat today?

Take a minute, close your eyes, visualize the ideal healthier you.
What do you look like?   What can you do?   How do you feel?

Describe your vision

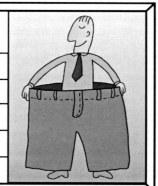

Acknowledge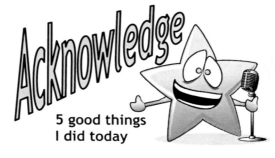

5 good things I did today

| 1 |
| 2 |
| 3 |
| 4 |
| 5 |

Day 82

DATE:

Five Deep Breaths

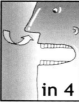 in 4

HOLD 4

 out 4

WAIT 4

Be Active

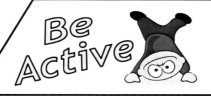

What physical activity did I do today ?

Raw Raw Raw

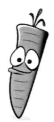

| Breakfast |
| Lunch |
| Dinner |

What raw fruits & veggies did I eat today?

 Exercise at least 30 minutes today. Make it continuous and enjoyable.

Once you start moving, keep moving for the entire time.

| 5 mins SLOW | 20 mins *FASTER* | 5 mins SLOW |

 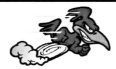

| What I did |
| How I felt |

Acknowledge

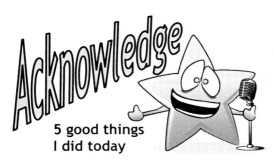

5 good things I did today

| 1 |
| 2 |
| 3 |
| 4 |
| 5 |

Day 83   DATE:

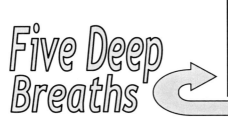 Five Deep Breaths

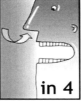 in 4   HOLD 4   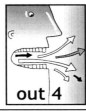 out 4   WAIT 4

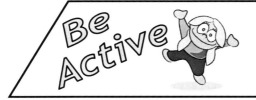 Be Active   **What physical activity did I do today ?**

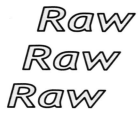 Raw Raw Raw

Breakfast	
Lunch	
Dinner	

What raw fruits & veggies did I eat today?

Appreciate Your Magnificent Body
List at least three things you appreciate about your body right now.

1	2	3

Pick one, and describe why you're grateful How do you feel about that?

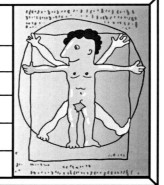

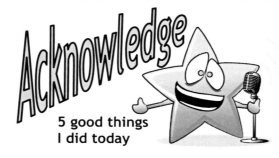 Acknowledge

5 good things I did today

1	
2	
3	
4	
5	

Day 84

DATE:

Five Deep Breaths

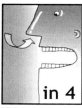 in 4

HOLD 4

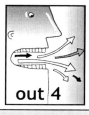 out 4

WAIT 4

Be Active

What physical activity did I do today?

Raw Raw Raw

Breakfast
Lunch
Dinner

What raw fruits & veggies did I eat today?

Exercise at least 30 minutes today.
Make it continuous and enjoyable.

Once you start moving,
keep moving for the entire time.

5 mins SLOW	20 mins *FASTER*	5 mins SLOW

What I did

How I felt

Acknowledge

5 good things I did today

1	
2	
3	
4	
5	

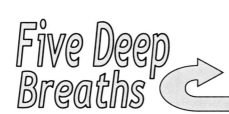

Day 85

DATE:

Five Deep Breaths

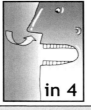 in 4   HOLD 4 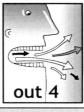 out 4   WAIT 4

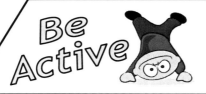 **Be Active**

What physical activity did I do today ?

Raw Raw Raw

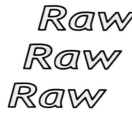

Breakfast	
Lunch	
Dinner	

What raw fruits & veggies did I eat today?

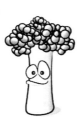

List five benefits of exercising regularly

1	
2	
3	
4	
5	

Acknowledge

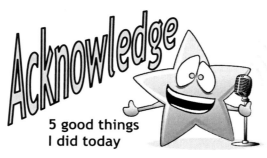

5 good things I did today

1	
2	
3	
4	
5	

Day 86

DATE:

Five Deep Breaths

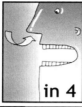 in 4   HOLD 4   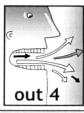 out 4   WAIT 4

Be Active

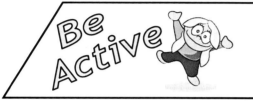

What physical activity did I do today ?

Raw Raw Raw

Breakfast
Lunch
Dinner

What raw fruits & veggies did I eat today?

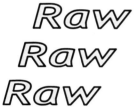

List five ways that anyone can make time for exercise

1	
2	
3	
4	
5	

Acknowledge

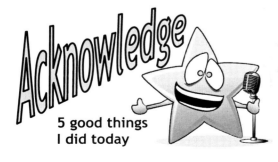

5 good things I did today

1	
2	
3	
4	
5	

Day 87

DATE:

Five Deep Breaths

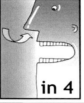

in 4

HOLD 4

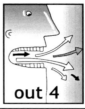

out 4

WAIT 4

Be Active

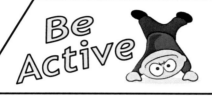

What physical activity did I do today ?

Raw Raw Raw

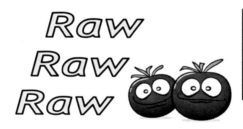

Breakfast
Lunch
Dinner

What raw fruits & veggies did I eat today?

Exercise at least 30 minutes today.
Make it continuous and enjoyable.

Once you start moving,
keep moving for the entire time.

| 5 mins SLOW | 20 mins *FASTER* | 5 mins SLOW |

 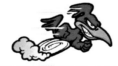

What I did
How I felt

Acknowledge

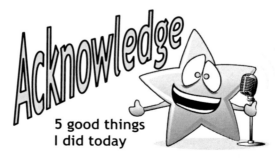

5 good things
I did today

1	
2	
3	
4	
5	

Day 88   DATE:

Five Deep Breaths

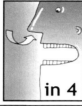 in 4   HOLD 4 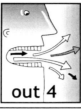 out 4   WAIT 4

Be Active
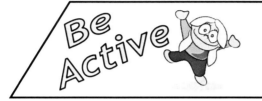

What physical activity did I do today ?

Raw Raw Raw
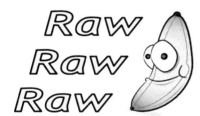

Breakfast	
Lunch	
Dinner	

What raw fruits & veggies did I eat today?

Take a minute, close your eyes, visualize the ideal healthier you.
What do you look like?   What can you do?   How do you feel?

Describe your vision

Acknowledge
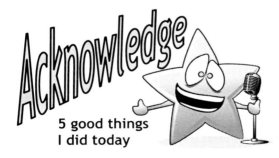

5 good things I did today

1	
2	
3	
4	
5	

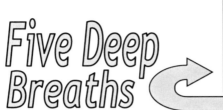

Five Deep Breaths

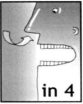 in 4

 HOLD 4

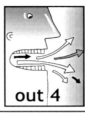 out 4

 WAIT 4

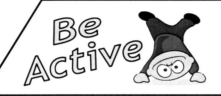

What physical activity did I do today?

Raw Raw Raw

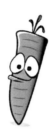

Breakfast	
Lunch	
Dinner	

What raw fruits & veggies did I eat today?

Exercise at least 30 minutes today.
Make it continuous and enjoyable.

Once you start moving,
keep moving for the entire time.

What I did
How I felt

5 mins SLOW	20 mins *FASTER*	5 mins SLOW

 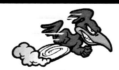

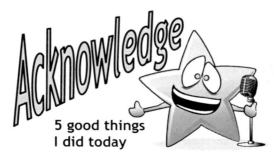

Acknowledge

5 good things
I did today

1	
2	
3	
4	
5	

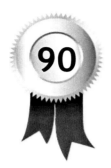

90

Date

Reflect on your Progress

Take a few minutes to flip back
through the pages of the last thirty days.

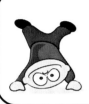 Over the last 30 days, what activities were the most fun,
and easiest to incorporate in to your life?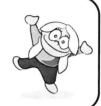

 What new fruits or vegetables did you experience over the last 30 days?
What value are you receiving from eating raw foods?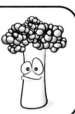

What benefits have you noticed from exercising regularly?
What are you enjoying most about your exercise routine?

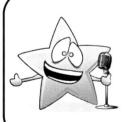 What have you learned about yourself over the last 30 days?

Outstanding...

You've done it.
Now, it's time to really celebrate.

Reevaluation

You have successfully completed the *Healthy Habit Former* 90 day, self directed action plan. Let's compare your present lifestyle habits with those you benchmarked 90 days ago.

I currently exercise

| never | occasionally | In a week: | 1 x | 2 x | 3 x | MORE |

What role does exercise have in determining how you feel overall?

| Not important | somewhat important | very important | essential |

What is your current attitude towards exercise?

| hate it | it's okay | enjoy it | love it |

I eat raw fruits and vegetables:

| never | occasionally | In a day: | 1 x | 2 x | 3 x | MORE |

I think raw fruits taste:

| disgusting | okay | good | delicious |

I think raw vegetables taste:

| disgusting | okay | good | delicious |

How would you describe your ability to calm and relax yourself?

| very difficult | I can sometimes | I can most times | I can anytime |

How do you feel about yourself and your current lifestyle?

| not happy | somewhat happy | pretty happy | fantastic |

Good job! Now flip back to the Benchmark on page 1.09
See which responses are different today from those of 90 days ago.

4.01

Healthy Habit Former

How to Proceed from Here

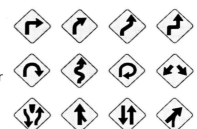

To maintain your current level of health, it is important to continue practicing your new habits. You can do this by simply beginning the program over at Day 1. You can either order a new *Healthy Habit Former,* or use some blank sheets of paper to record your activities. By doing this you will sustain the health and fitness level you have achieved.

I have a gift for you. I reward commitment, and you have shown tremendous commitment by completing your 90-day action plan. To celebrate this effort, I am offering you one free twenty-minute telephone coaching session. This is ideal if you are ready to take your fitness to the next level. Together we'll discuss an approach that's right for you. Email me to set up your session at Astrid@SynergenixFitness.com

I look forward to hearing about your successes.

In good health,

Astrid

Astrid Whiting
Synergenix Fitness

> *One of the greatest discoveries a man makes,*
> *one of his greatest surprises,*
> *is to find he can do what he was afraid he couldn't do.*
>
> Henry Ford

Need a speaker for your next event

We love to talk about fitness. Astrid is available for interviews, keynotes, and to conduct workshops and seminars.

Let's discuss a fitness and health topic that is right for your group.

Contact her at Astrid@SynergenixFitness.com or (250) 888-4099

Achieve Your Vibrant Health Body

Want to reach their fitness goals without working harder?
Wish you habitually made healthy choices instinctively?

This 26-minute self-hypnosis visualization audio CD harnesses the awesome power of your subconscious mind on your journey to optimal health.

Listen to this, and you will
- *Intuitively make healthier food choices*
  that will satisfy your body's nutritional needs
- *Visualize your ideal body*
  to automatically ignite your drive to exercise
- *Escape from daily stressors*
  to rejuvenate your body and mind

The Personal Growth Activator

Ever promise yourself you'd improve your life?
What happened to that goal?

This 26-minute self-hypnosis audio CD is designed to supplement personal growth initiatives by helping you to take your action plan from concept to execution.

Listen to this, and you will
- *Activate your personal growth plan*
  to achieve your desired outcomes
- *Stay excited about your goals*
  to sustain momentum and focus
- *Complete what you've started*
  and feel proud of your personal success

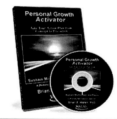

Personal and Post Re-hab Training

Achieving your fitness goals requires both mental and physical commitment. At *Synergenix Fitness*, our one-on-one training is custom-designed to meet the needs of your body and mind. The process begins with a private consultation. Your certified trainer will take into account your current health, fitness level, mind-set, and lifestyle to design a program that meets your objectives.

Body Composition Assessments

Want to track your progress towards your health goals?
Have you finally realized your scale provides useless information?
Then it's time to get the information that really matters.

Body Composition Assessments done using bioelectrical impedance technology provide the most relevant information for determining overall health:
- ♦ Percentage of body fat
- ♦ Percentage of lean mass
- ♦ Total pounds of lean mass
- ♦ Total pounds of fat
- ♦ Hydration levels
- ♦ Basal metabolic rate

4.03

This precise, science-based assessment is accurate, simple and non-invasive.